To Jerri

Best of health

To you.

All of the food pictures in this book are real, prepared and taken by Peter in his kitchen, before being enjoyed by his family.

Peter K. MS, PT

Shop. Cook. Eat.

Eating Healthy in an Unhealthy World

7 Rules for Choosing Real, Delicious, Sustainable Foods

Back to Nature Books

Peter K

Since he was a young boy, Peter has always gravitated toward the natural world. However, due to unfortunate events early in his life, he found himself unhealthy and overweight. Today he loves to grow his own food, cook from scratch, and is a student of the local, sustainable food movement. During his personal health journey he has become an International Health Coach, Nutritionist, Physical Therapist, Speaker and Author. He's also been called, "The Missing Link", in corporate wellness. As an expert for the media, he has appeared on ABC, QVC, FOX, MSN, TLC, Blogtalkradio and in *Fitness Magazine*. He's the author of *Shop, Cook, Eat*, *The Live Better Journal*, and *The Core Energy Program*. He's the creator of the 5 Minutes to Fitness+ Program & Online Club, a revolutionary lifestyle program for achieving optimal health, which has been featured on QVC and FOX. His clients include: celebrities, "Fortune 100" companies, non-profit organizations and individuals who have made incredible changes in their work, life, health and happiness

Notice

All information presented by Peter K Fitness, LLC is for education purposes only. The material is not intended to be a substitute for medical counseling. You should always consult with your physician before starting any health program. If any of the suggestions in this program contradict your physician's advice, be sure to consult your doctor before proceeding. If you have any medical conditions or issues, you should consult with your doctor immediately.

P.S. Make sure your health professional engages in a healthy lifestyle.

P.P.S. Be cautious when taking health advice from pharmaceutical and industrial food companies.

Peter K Fitness, LLC
shopcookeatrealfood.com
peterkfitness.com
contact@peterkfitness.com
877-364-7383

For my family,

Dana, Anna, Emma, & Alexander

The best reasons to shop, cook, and eat healthy

In Memory of SDR
Too soon my friend...

Acknowledgements

Thank you to Wendell Berry, Joan Gussow, Alice Waters, Elliot Coleman, Michael Pollan, Joel Salatin, Dan Barber, and those who came before them. And thank you to the farmers, bakers, butchers, fishmongers, fermenters, and others who preserve food traditions, often regardless of personal financial consequences.

A Note to the reader

You'll notice some of my advice is repeated throughout this book. That's to help reiterate the simple, but important concepts of eating healthier and to allow you to skip around in the book. Read it how you wish and enjoy every dish.

Wise Proverb

Eat More Honeymoon Salads

Lettuce Alone, With No Dressing

Table Of Contents

Preface (Cheat Sheet)

3 Steps For Eating Healthier, Almost Anywhere, Anytime

My hope is that you'll read this entire book because it's essentially a summary of 23 years of nutrition knowledge, blended with my love of growing, cooking and eating real food. But, I know you're busy, so start by reading this cheat sheet. The best foods have these qualities:

Whole, Wild, Organic, Fresh, Local, Ethnic, Seasonal

First **Seek Whole Foods:** Real foods in or close to their natural state, 5 ingredients or less, recognizable, pronounceable, no artificial additives, typically don't come in boxes or wrappers, and your great, great grandma would recognize them. They're typically more nutritious, flavorful, fiber rich, have healthier fats, and no refined sugars. They're the foundation of healthy eating and come from farms, the wild, or water. *Vegetables, Fruit, Whole Grains, Nuts, Seeds, *Animal Protein*

Then **Eat The Seasons:** Eat seasonal fresh, frozen, or naturally preserved foods. More nutritious, flavorful, typically local whole foods, *sustainable, support local businesses, decrease pollution/global warming, offer variety, and connect us to the earth. Search for seasonal foods where you live. Come from gardens, farms, farmer's markets, **CSA's and better grocery stores. Includes frozen when fresh, naturally preserved, and fermented foods.

Also **Look For Organic, Grass-Fed & Pastured:** Generally more nutritious, flavorful, sustainable, and may be local. Foods labeled organic by the USDA or other certifying body, cannot contain pesticides, herbicides, fungicides, antibiotics, growth hormones, or genetically modified organisms (****GMOs).

Choose organic fruit, vegetables, grains, chicken, turkey, pork, & lamb

Choose grass-fed (pastured) beef and bison

Organic Note: Sometimes local farms are not certified organic because it's an expensive process. Ask them if they use organic, biodynamic, sustainable practices. Chances are they do and we should support them.

*Animal Protein: Grass-Fed/Pastured Sustainably raised cows & bison, live on pastures and are free to graze on grass & other natural feed, higher in omega-3s, and less fat & calories. These animals live natural lives, eating foods they were meant to eat. Pastured, Grass-Fed, and Grass Finished mean the same thing. These animals are healthier than conventionally raised animals

**Sustainable: Involving methods that do not completely use up or destroy natural resources.

***CSA (Community Supported Agriculture): Basically you sign up with a local farm or group and receive fresh, local, seasonal produce and other local products bi-monthly, or monthly. Check out - http://www.localharvest.org, or shop at a local farm or farmer's market.

****GMOs (Genetically Modified Foods): These foods have been genetically modified. Many contain pesticides and other substances/qualities that yield quantity, but lack nutritional quality. If a food is not local or organic, there is an 80–90% chance it contains GMOs. GMOs harm the soil and cause tumors in lab animals. All certified organic foods are GMO free. Ask your food suppliers if their foods contain GMOs.

80/20 Eating Rule: I've found that if I eat the foods in this book 80% of the time, and indulge the remaining 20%, I stay healthy, enjoy food, and look and feel great.

Motivation: I've observed that the healthiest, most fulfilled people are the ones who have compelling reasons for doing what they do, like eating great. I've also noticed that they consistently eat the foods in this book. They don't diet.

Introduction

Introduction

Conundrum – If your food didn't come from a farm, the wild, or water, can it still be called food?

Eating Healthy in an Unhealthy World

If someone were to ask me the best thing they can do to be healthy, I'd tell them, based on my personal and professional experience, studying the world's healthiest people, and most importantly, my desire to help my three children eat healthy in an unhealthy world, to:

"Eat real food."

This book will help you do that.

Peter K

Why and How I Wrote This Book

Has anyone ever told you to do something you knew was good for you, but you didn't, because you don't like being told what to do? Me too. I dislike when I'm lectured to, so I have tried not to do that to you in this book. Eating healthy is personal, exciting, and for many of us, somewhat difficult.

Besides relating nutritional prudence, my desire in writing this book was to share my personal experiences as a fellow foodie, attempting to shop, cook, and eat healthy in an unhealthy world, while also trying to fit into a pair of jeans - let's be honest.

In these pages you'll find what I view as exciting food trends & choices, as well as insights from 23 years of my own health journey. To my surprise, I've learned considerably more by talking to farmers, reading books, gardening, and cooking for my own children in my own kitchen, than I ever did sitting in nutrition lectures in school. This is what I've learned:

"One of the best things you can do for your health is to shop for, cook, and eat real food, made simply from scratch, several times per week."

My goal is to show you how to do that. In the following pages I share bites of my everyday health journey, relate real food stories, how to find and cook the best foods, and, best of all, how to eat them. I hope you'll enjoy the recipes, and that they'll tempt you back into the kitchen, or at least view cooking from a new perspective.

Feel free to skip ahead to *Rule 1- Whole Foods*, and start learning about the healthiest foods. But if you want to learn how Michele, along with the rest of us, can eat better, without sacrificing taste or flavor, read the next page.

2

Meet Michele - You may know someone like her, intimately.

"I want to lose weight and eat healthy, but I'm too busy, not sure what to choose, and I love food!" **Michele - busy professional, full-time job, wife, mother of 2**

The Problem

Michele, along with about 90% of the people I meet, are not eating healthfully; dining on processed and fast foods. This is not a judgment, but rather an observation. Of the remaining 10% who believe they are eating healthy, 9% consume some sort of shake, supplement, or synthetic food that was designed in a lab and contains unrecognizable ingredients. About 1% of people eat the way that is described in this book. They are typically the healthiest people. Soon you'll see it's not difficult to eat like them, most of the time - You don't have to be perfect.

"Whenever you find yourself on the side of the majority, it is time to pause and reflect." - Mark Twain

Michele's Dilemma

Michele begged for a diet with the best foods for weight loss, and better health. She confessed she really didn't know what was healthy because of confusing media messages. She also wanted to know if the energy bars and protein shakes she regularly consumed, instead of meals, were healthy. On inspection, they each contained more than 15 ingredients, most unrecognizable. She had her answer.

Terroir (ter wahr): When a food tastes like the place it came from. Example; Wine grapes from Chardonnay region soil. Grape flavored protein shake from...a lab?

Why is it So Hard to Eat Healthy?

Why do many of us, like Michele, think we need someone to tell us what's healthy, how much to eat, what to avoid? Why are so many of us struggling with weight and illness? Why are our children getting adult diseases younger, and in alarming numbers? And, most frustrating, why is eating so darn guilt ridden?

I've observed that the answers can be linked to two simple, yet inextricably linked facts:

Fact # 1

Most of us, like Michele, do not live on farms anymore. We don't grow the foods we eat, and we don't always buy fresh, whole foods from the local farmer's markets traditionally found around the world. Most of us aren't choosing, preparing, cooking, and eating the seasonal, local, ethnic, whole foods that our great, great, grandma ate. This is the *root* of the problem (Pun intended).

Fact #2

We find ourselves in this peculiar dilemma primarily because of something extraordinary that's going on that you may not be aware of. Because we're so busy, and far removed from our food sources, many of us are getting our meals, as well as our nutrition advice, from industrial food companies that promote the new four food groups: **trans fat**, **refined sugar**, **über salt** and **artificial additives** (non-traditional, non-local foods).

Not that there's anything inherently bad about the first 3 - fat, sugar, & salt - in their whole, natural forms, or all of them, once in awhile. It's just that for the first time in history, someone else (big business) is growing, preparing, and cooking

4

food for us, the majority of the time, using a cocktail of said ingredients as their base. That's where things go wrong: think obesity, cancer, diabetes, heart disease, high blood pressure, and the like.

We live lives that are technologically advanced, but, ironically, nutritionally disadvantaged. We may live far from where our food is grown, out of touch with how it gets to us, and how that impacts our health, and the earth. During the course of our day we may never step on grass or dirt (severing our connection to the earth), we may eat processed food while driving, or staring at a screen, and when we're too busy to eat, we're tempted to reach for energy that comes in a bottle and claims to last for 5 hours. It's no wonder we're so tired, struggling with weight, and feeling the effects of inferior foods and chronic stress: anxious, depressed, unmotivated, bloated, tired, unhappy.

> **Feeling Bad?** - *If you persistently feel fatigued, "achy", bloated, or depressed, you may be negatively affected by processed foods, or you may have a food allergy, intolerance, or sensitivity. Keep a food journal, or ask your (healthy) doctor for a blood test, and start exploring the foods in this book.*

The Solution (Yes, There Is Good News)

Instead of prescribing Michele yet another diet, and knowing she wasn't ready to start farming, I wanted her to be empowered to eat healthy almost anywhere, anytime; simply and easily, and for the rest of her life. To help her, I made a list of the healthiest foods based on the soundest nutrition wisdom and traditional food practices, including the foods I

5

consistently choose for my family. That's when I noticed that all these foods had the following in common: they were in or close to their whole form, and from traditional food sources, such as; **smaller farms, the wild, oceans and rivers**.

I started to categorize these foods by their qualities and created rules for finding them. This made it easy for Michele, or anyone else, to walk into a grocery store, restaurant, or food source, and simply choose the best foods. This is where WWOFLES (waffles) came from.

What Are WWOFLES?

Pronounced "waffles", WWOFLES is an acronym for:

Whole, Wild, Organic, Fresh, Local, Ethnic, Seasonal

WWOFLES is a simple way to remember how to choose healthy food, almost anywhere, almost anytime. The food qualities in WWOFLES make up the 7 rules for finding the healthiest foods that the healthiest people have consistently eaten throughout history.

These foods also happen to taste great, are more and more available, and are part of a food revolution founded on local, sustainable, community-focused foods; grown, harvested, and prepared traditionally; and centered on quality, not quantity. This book, using these 7 rules, will show you how to find and prepare them.

> ***Note:*** *I've always been skeptical of diets, fads and miracle supplements. However, I've always found value in strategies that are easy to remember, effective, and based on natural food rules. That's WWOFLES.*

6

For the skeptic, here is a fun example of how Michele can use WWOFLES anywhere, anytime to eat healthy in the most improbable setting. Try this your self.

Step 1. Enter McDonalds

Step 2. Leave

Step 3. Find WWOFLES foods

Search for 2-3 WWOFLES qualities at every meal and you'll be eating healthier.

For example, if you're in a deli, restaurant, or market, think WWOFLES and order a *Fresh Salad with Organic dressing: Lettuce, tomato, cucumber, red onion, & organic dressing. This salad consists of 3 WWOFLES qualities: Whole, Organic, and Fresh foods*

The diagram below gives you a visual to make the concept clearer.

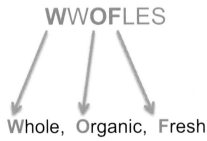

WWOFLES

Whole, Organic, Fresh

Lettuce, tomato, cucumber, red onion, organic dressing

NOTE: I hope it's obvious; we shouldn't look to fast food as a healthy food source because the quality of the food is generally poor. In fact, Michele's admitted that she wants to avoid, or at least limit, processed and fast food. She could easily pick up take-out on her way home for her kids after a long day. It's certainly cheaper (when did cheap food become the desired norm for our children?) but what price is her family really paying: think poor health and environmental damage from harmful food growing practices.

We now know the following: when companies cook for us, as a rule, they typically do not use the best quality ingredients when they "design" their meals. This fact generally makes the processed and fast food industry a poor *quality* food source. Studies now confirm what we've intuited; when we eat poor quality processed foods, we get sick. This is a poor recipe for health.

Observation- *Real food is grown, rather than designed.*

Good Quality Food Vs. Poor Quality Food

What's encouraging is some of us are already choosing better quality foods. However, it's still alarming to observe that many more of us, especially our children, are eating poor quality foods everyday, including pseudo-healthy foods; shakes, supplements and prepared foods. There is also a theoretical claim that industrialized food can feed more people more cheaply. But, we're finding that's not the case, and there's a cost to be paid in the form of poor health and environmental consequences. Read *The Omnivore's Dilemma.*

That leaves us with the fact that most of us want to eat healthier, but don't know where to start. Here are two comparisons to help us make better choices. One involves cows, and the other salads. The facts of these side-by-side comparisons are known to some, and alarming to others. They make it obvious which foods we'd rather bite into, and serve to our children.

Let's compare Ingrid the industrial cow to Patty the pastured cow.

Adapted from Michael Pollan's, The Omnivore's Dilemma.

Industrial Animals:

Today's modern, industrialized farms raise unhealthy animals. Cows, chickens and pigs are fed GMO corn and soy. This unnatural diet makes the animals sick, requiring the use of medications and pharmaceuticals like antibiotics. The animals live in their own excrement due to overcrowding, creating lakes of toxic waste in the form of manure that's too polluted to be used as fertilizer. You and I eventually eat this meat and it makes us sick and resistant to antibiotics. This is not a sustainable system.

Pastured Animals:

Good quality food comes from traditional farms that respect and support nature's cycles; on **Biodynamic** farms, **pastured** cows eat grass (grass-fed), which they were intended to eat, so they're healthier. Their manure spreads more grass seed and fertilizes it at the same time. Chickens then eat the parasites and grubs in the cow's manure, preventing the spread of disease and making the chickens healthier. The animals are healthier, providing us with healthier food. The cycle is repeated and is self-sustaining.

Pastured animals are labeled, "Pastured", "Grass-Fed", or "Grass-Finished" and are more and more available.

Now let's compare a poor quality salad with a good quality salad. If this side-by-side comparison doesn't speak to you then this book may not be for you.

Poor Quality Salad - (Fast Food Salad)
Ingredients typically found in most fast foods

Lettuce: picked un-ripe for long travel (wastes fossil fuel), lack of taste, poor nutrition, contains pesticides.

Tomatoes: genetic mutations bred for uniformity, contains pesticides, picked un-ripe, lacks the flavor and nutrition of an in-season, local tomato.

Cheese: contains hormones (cancer causing) & antibiotics, processed, artificially flavored and colored, ingredients, and cows fed GMOs (corn and soy).

Chicken: fed GMO corn and soy (non traditional feed), given antibiotics, and live in their own feces.

Dressing: processed, artificially sweetened, preservatives added, and can include: (This is an actual ingredient list; do you recognize all these foods?)

> WATER, VINEGAR, HIGH FRUCTOSE CORN SYRUP, CORN SYRUP, SALT, CONTAINS LESS THAN 2% OF PARMESAN CHEESE* (PART-SKIM MILK, CHEESE CULTURE, SALT, ENZYMES), GARLIC, ONION JUICE, WHEY, PHOSPHORIC ACID, XANTHAN GUM, POTASSIUM SORBATE AND CALCIUM DISODIUM EDTA AS PRESERVATIVES, YEAST EXTRACT, SPICE, RED BELL PEPPERS*, LEMON JUICE CONCENTRATE, GARLIC*, BUTTERMILK*, CARAMEL COLOR, SODIUM PHOSPHATE, ENZYMES, OLEORESIN PAPRIKA. *DRIED.

Now lets compare that salad with a good quality salad using the WWOFLES concept.

Good Quality Salad- Includes 5 WWOFLES ingredients;Whole, Fresh, Local, Organic, Seasonal

➡ *Lettuce:* local, in-season, crisp, nutritious, sweet, delicious, pesticide free, sustainably grown.

➡ *Tomatoes*: local, in season, picked ripe (full nutrition and flavor), pesticide free, no genetic mutations, no pesticides.

➡ *Cheese* (optional): organic, artisanal, made with real cultures, no hormones, antibiotics or GMOs. *Instead of cheese* - beans, eggs, wild salmon, almonds for protein.

➡ *Chicken:* fed organic feed, more omega-3s, humanely & sustainably raised and beneficial to the environment

➡ *Dressing:* Balsamic Dijon Vinaigrette p. 67. Ingredients - balsamic vinegar, Dijon mustard, olive oil, pinch of salt; that's it.

Tip- If a food is labeled Organic, it cannot contain GMOs. (Genetically Modified Organisms)

Can't Get Motivated to Eat Healthier?

When it comes to motivation, I have observed that those who have a personally compelling reason to eat healthier are the ones who are the most motivated. What's your personally compelling reason to make better food choices? I suggest making it more exciting than just losing weight. Do you want to look great, have more energy, be a better role model for your kids, or run a marathon? Whatever your reason, make it exciting!

Also, there's a phenomenon that occurs when you eat WWOFLES foods, that will help keep you motivated. Your craving for processed foods laden with fat, sugar, salt, and synthetic additives will decrease. In fact, processed foods will start to taste artificial to you. Your mouth will discern the additives in your food, and your mind will gradually shun them from your repertoire. It typically takes a couple of weeks for this to happen, but it will happen.

Also, those who eat WWOFLES quality foods will assure you; you don't have to sacrifice great taste for health. When you eat the foods showcased in this book you'll experience foods with exceptional flavor that taste like what they are, are packed with nutrition, and are satisfying. My experience has been that you'll actually start to crave the foods in the recipes and recommendations throughout this book, including vegetables, for those with an aversion.

> **OBSERVATION**- *I'm convinced children won't "eat their veggies" because they may never have had "real" ones: grown locally, organically, picked ripe, in-season, simply prepared, and accompanied by a miraculous story about their journeys from seed to plate. This makes a carrot more appetizing, and just tastes better.*

You Don't Have to Count Calories

When you eat the foods in this book you don't have to count calories, worry if you're getting enough fiber, or diet ever again. That's because you'll be eating the best quality foods that are more nourishing, filling and satisfying.

Doesn't Organic Cost More?

There's a perception that healthy food costs more. In many cases, it appears to. I advise people it's a personal choice. I've learned this from my food mentors; there are other costs to be paid when we don't seek better foods- like poor health and damage to the environment. If you shop for local, seasonal foods at farms and farmers markets, you'll very often find they are more affordable. Do your best.

The 80/20 Eating Rule

One last bit of encouraging news, you don't have to eat perfectly all the time. In my experience, if you eat the foods in this book just 80% of the time, you'll be getting the health benefits, including disease prevention, and you'll look and feel younger. For example, I've observed that if you eat a great breakfast and lunch, you can indulge a little at dinner, say with some wine, or a reasonable dessert. Or, if you've eaten great all week, you can indulge during one meal on the weekend without sabotaging your efforts. The healthiest people eat well 80% of the time (the foods in this book), and indulge 20% of the time.

Now, enjoy the following pages as eating pleasure, health, and earth stewardship, finally and favorably merge. When we realize we can both love food and eat healthy at the same time, while doing our part to preserve the earth, we are giving our children a sustainable gift.

Bon Appetit!

Rule 1: Choose Whole Foods

"The whole is MORE than the sum of its PARTS"
- Aristotle

Is Pizza a Whole Food?

When I first told my friend the **W** in **WWOFLES** stands for whole, she cheered, "As in a whole pizza!!??" "Nice try", I said. "It means whole, as in whole foods, like a carrot." She looked disappointed.

Pizza can be a whole food meal if it's made with whole, real, ingredients like; whole wheat flour, whole cheese (milk, natural enzymes, salt) and whole tomato sauce (tomatoes, basil, oil, salt) without artificial preservatives, stabilizers, or flavor enhancers like Cellulose Powder, Potassium Sorbate, and whatever peculiar additives food companies sneak into pizza.

Back to carrots: Carrots, I informed my friend, are healthiest, and most flavorful in variations of their whole form: sliced and roasted, julienned over salad, or simply enjoyed raw. If you've never tried a local, organic, in-season carrot, you've never tasted the incredible sweetness of a carrot. They've been likened to candy.

The Best Eating Starts Here

Whole foods are the foundation of healthy eating. They generally look like what they are, are void of artificial additives, and are rich in nutrients and flavor. When we consume them whole we're most likely getting the most nutritional benefit. You'll find them with little or no packaging and usually without labels; think produce aisles, farmer's markets, butcher and seafood counters, gardens, and farms. Also, whole foods can be combined with other whole foods to create whole food meals, like pizza.

When big companies process foods, or separate out healthy components, like fiber, there's no guarantee we're still getting a health benefit, regardless of what their marketing tells us. Beta-carotene and fiber, found naturally in carrots, work best together in our bodies. When we put them in a pill or designer drink we're not guaranteed the same health benefit. Some companies attempt to create "super foods" this way, but I think that's redundant. Just eat the whole food.

Whole, Wild, Organic, Fresh, Local, Ethnic, Seasonal

WWOFLES

Whole Foods

Whole Foods – REAL FOODS, in or close to their natural state, have recognizable ingredients, are minimally processed (typically don't come in boxes or wrappers) and generally provide you with their full health benefit. They're the foundation of healthy eating. Base all meals on whole foods. *Includes:* Fresh, Frozen, Canned, Preserved and Fermented*

Examples: Fruit, Vegetables, Legumes (Beans), Whole Grains (e.g. Quinoa, Millet), Nuts, Seeds, Meat, Fish, Poultry, and Game

*Best Choices***:** Carrots, Broccoli, Apples, Beans, Oats, Sardines, Quinoa, Chicken, Sunflower Seeds, Eggs, Spinach, Sweet Potatoes, Pickles, Frozen Peas, Fruit Jams, Canned Tomatoes

Recipe Suggestions: Gourmet French Veggies (next page), Fig, Prosciutto, Gorgonzola Pizza (p. 89), Kale Soup with San Marzano Tomatoes (p. 69), Greek Village Salad (p. 55), Mu Shu Chicken with Lettuce Wraps (p. 71)

*A Note on Fermented Foods: Wild yeasts and bacteria, which cause fermentation, partially break down foods making them more digestible and nutritious, impart a unique flavor and preserve foods. Includes: **Bread, Pickles, Wine, Vinegar, Beer, Sauerkraut, Kombucha, Miso, Tempeh, Cheese, Yogurt.** Look for those without artificial additives.

*The Best Whole Grains***:** The healthiest whole grains are labeled "100% stone ground".

Eating "whole foods" does not mean you have to eat the peel of an orange - Real question.

Whole Food Recipe

Gourmet French Vegetables

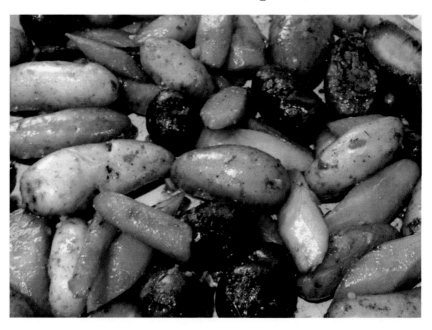

I love veggies now like I never did as a child. Maybe it's because I grow them in my yard. I've never tasted a carrot like the ones I pick from my garden; in season, fresh, and simply prepared. They're al dente and sweet.

This recipe comes from my mentor Jacques Pepin. The vegetables are cooked on the stovetop, are ready in minutes, taste spectacular, and will make you look like a French chef in the kitchen.

For all recipes in this book, I encourage you to buy organic veggies, preferably from a local source like a farmer's market. What you get in the large supermarkets are species cultivated for production, not flavor or nutrition.

Love to read about food? I recommend Jacques Pepin's memoir, ***The Apprentice: My Life in the Kitchen***

Gourmet French Vegetables

Serves 4-5

What You'll Need

carrots, 3 large, peeled and cleaned, sliced into ¼ inch lengths on the bias (angled)

heirloom fingerling potatoes, 10 – 11 small

red onions, 1 large, halved then sliced into slivers

garlic, 3 cloves, chopped

vegetable or chicken stock, 1/2 cup

olive oil, extra virgin, expeller (cold) pressed, to taste

thyme, 1 tablespoon fresh , or 1 teaspoon dried

salt & pepper to taste

To Prepare

1 Heat a large stainless steel skillet to medium (you can use a nonstick as well). Drizzle with oil and drop in the onions. Cook for 2 minutes, stirring often.

2 Then add the carrots, potatoes, garlic and seasonings, cook 2 more minutes, and add the vegetable stock. Stir, turn heat to low and cover.

3 Cook for 15-20 minutes, checking and stirring often. Cook until veggies are fork tender, then remove lid, turn heat to medium high and cook until browned (caramelized) and almost all the liquid is evaporated. Salt & pepper to taste. Serve warm with a final drizzle of olive oil. Bon Appetit!

Serving Suggestions

For the best flavor, serve these veggies in summer and fall, when they're in season. Get creative and add your favorite root vegetables. Jacques Pepin serves variations of this with his famous Beef Bourguignon (see recipe p. 72). You can also try it with fish, chicken, lamb, or as a main dish.

Rule 2: Choose Wild Foods

"In Wildness is the preservation of the world"
- Henry David Thoreau

Wild Things and "Chicken Eatin' Fish"

My local fishmonger carries farmed and wild salmon, when the latter is in season. The wild salmon costs double, but I always choose it. He whispers in my ear to buy the farmed because it's cheaper, available year-round, and he's not convinced that wild is any healthier. I respectfully but confidently tell him why I believe wild is a better choice:

> *Wild fish and game are leaner, more flavorful, do not contain pesticides, hormones or antibiotics and are typically healthier than farmed fish and conventional (non-organic) livestock. For example, studies show that wild salmon contains more beneficial omega-3s, and other nutrients as compared to farmed salmon. They are also inherently stronger (healthier) having to survive in nature, which means when we eat them, we benefit.*

Disturbingly, some farmed fish are fed wheat, soy, and yes, chicken. The thought of eating fish that was fed chicken is disturbing, and some say the fish tastes like, well, chicken. Question modern food growing practices that seem bizarre and counterproductive, like aqua farming which raises concerns regarding illness, the use of antibiotics, and the disruption of the natural balance of ecosystems.

Why Wild Foods Are Healthier

Wild fish, animals, and plants live a more natural life cycle, eat foods they're designed to eat, have to fight for their survival making them healthier, and, if harvested in a responsible way, can be environmentally sustainable.

Also, wild foods, like vegetables and fruit, as well as fish and animals, have more nutrition than conventionally grown foods. "Conventional" means not wild or organic. Conventional is a red flag to me indicating the food is most likely genetically modified or grown in a monoculture (picture acres of just corn or soybeans which deplete soil, invite disease, and decrease the flavor of foods). Live on the wild side and choose wild foods.

Whole, Wild, Organic, Fresh, Local, Ethnic, Seasonal

WWOFLES

Wild Foods

Wild Foods - Plants and animals that live in the wild. They live a more natural lifecycle and can provide better nutrition because they fight for their survival, increasing their antioxidant levels and other beneficial qualities.

Examples: Fish, Fruit, Salad Greens, Game, Mushrooms (trusted source), Rice, Honey, *Wild Fermentation Foods: Pickles, Sauerkraut, Bread, Alcohol, Cheese, Vinegar.

Best Choices: Salmon, Shiitake Mushrooms, Dandelion Greens, Blueberries, Crab Apples, Arugula, Cherries, Boar, Venison, Rabbit, Beer, Wine, Cheese, Sourdough Bread.

Recipe Suggestions: Teriyaki Grilled Wild Salmon (next page), Wild Salmon over Spinach (p. 77), Arugula Salad, Garlic & Oil Sautéed Dandelion Greens, Wild Boar Sausage with Sauerkraut, Wild Salad Greens with Gorgonzola and Balsamic Vinegar

Great bread has 4 ingredients: flour, water, salt, and wild yeast/bacteria (starter). It's called sourdough bread.

Bitter is better: a bitter flavor means more phytonutrients making foods resilient to pests, and healthier for us.

Wild Fermentation Foods: Wild yeast and bacteria are used to make bread, wine, sauerkraut, kimchee, pickles, cheese and other fermented foods. These foods impart a health benefit from the fermentation process, which partially breaks down food making it more nutritious and digestible, introduces beneficial microbes into your gut, enhances flavor, and naturally preserves foods. Look for "wild fermentation", "natural starter", and "live active cultures" on labels.

Wild Food Recipe

Teriyaki Grilled Wild Salmon

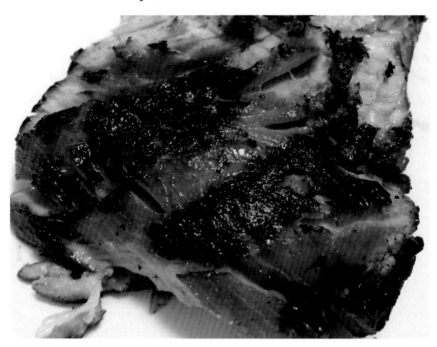

I think one of the best things in life is eating something delicious that also happens to be exceptionally healthy. Salmon is one of those foods, but only when it's wild. If you're eating for health, don't waste your money and good intentions on farmed salmon. It's just not as healthy.

I like to buy my wild salmon from my local fishmonger. (Support your local food purveyors) I like a filet with the skin on. You can discard it after cooking or enjoy its charred crunch. The teriyaki in this recipe masks any "fishy" taste.

Fish to avoid: Farmed Salmon, Swordfish, Chilean Sea Bass

Want to learn more about wild fermentation? Check out http://www.wildfermentation.com/

Teriyaki Grilled Wild Salmon

1 serving is 3–5 ounces, (deck of cards, palm of hand)

What You'll Need

wild salmon, filet, 3-5 ounces per person

teriyaki marinade, my favorite is "Soy Vay Teriyaki"

Ziploc bag

To Prepare

1 Place the fish in the plastic bag, pour in the marinade, enough to cover, and let sit in the fridge for 10 - 20 minutes, (no longer or the fish can get "mushy" and start to cook).

2 Preheat your BBQ grill to medium/high.

3 When hot, wipe grates with oil and place salmon skin side up on the grill. Cook for 3-5 minutes. Flip and cook for another 3-5 minutes or until it easily flakes under the pressure of your finger and the flesh is firm but moist. Serve warm and enjoy!

Bon Appetit!

Serving Suggestions

Try serving over salad greens, or garlic & oil sautéed spinach or kale, alongside quinoa, or with a baked sweet potato. I love grilling it, but you can also try broiling this recipe, or poach the salmon in a wine and dill bath.

Ask your fishmonger for other wild fish and seafood favorites like shrimp, lemon sole, scallops, sardines, cod, and haddock.

Rule 3: Choose Organic Foods

"Organic Oreos are not a health food"
- Michael Pollan

What's The Deal? Is Organic Better?

My friend's husband is skeptical about organics. He speculates it's a loose set of voluntary standards that allow growers to charge more, with little or no improvement in taste or nutritional benefit. He asks, "How do you know you're really getting organic, or that it means anything anyway?"

It's a fair question. I shared with him the organic standards below, then told him, "I know when I buy organic there's a good chance it's healthier and better for the earth. I know when I don't, my children are eating food that is not as healthy and most likely unsustainable." Sometimes you have to have faith.

Organically labeled foods cannot contain **pesticides, herbicides, and fungicides**. They're also **free of hormones & antibiotics and cannot be genetically modified**. Organic farming practices are sustainable because they include crop diversity and rotation that doesn't deplete the soil of nutrients.

Note: Your local farmer may be following organic standards but may not be organically certified because it's an expensive process. Get to know the people you buy your food from. Also, "**pastured**" is a practice that goes beyond organic. Look for pastured beef and bison. It's tastier, healthier, and sustainable.

US Government Organic guidelines:

Organic crops. The USDA organic seal verifies that irradiation, sewage sludge, synthetic fertilizers, prohibited pesticides, herbicides and fungicides, and genetically modified organisms were not used. And that the producers were certified by the USDA (United States Department of Agriculture) as upholding organic standards.

Organic livestock. The USDA organic seal verifies that producers meet animal health and welfare standards, did not use antibiotics or growth hormones, used 100% organic feed, and provided animals with access to the outdoors.

Organic multi-ingredient foods. The USDA organic seal verifies that the product has 95% or more certified organic content. If the label claims that it was made with specified organic ingredients, you can be sure that those specific ingredients are certified organic.

Whole, Wild, Organic, Fresh, Local, Ethnic, Seasonal

WWOFLES

Organic Foods

Organic Foods - Are labeled by the USDA or other certifying body. Organic foods cannot contain pesticides, herbicides, fungicides, antibiotics, growth hormones, or genetically modified organisms (GMOs). They are generally more nutritious, flavorful, and beneficial for the environment.

Examples: Fruit, Vegetables, Whole Grains, Nuts, Seeds, Dairy/Animal Products.

Caution: These contain the highest pesticide levels when **non-organic**; Strawberries, Apples, Spinach, Grapes, Bell Peppers, Potatoes, Celery, Peaches, Hot Peppers.

Recipe Suggestions: Blueberries & Eggs (next page), Bean, Corn, & Avocado Salad (p. 85), Chicken Fajitas with Homemade Guacamole (p. 83), BBQ Sauce Burgers (p. 81), Skirt Steak over Garden Greens with Tahini and Hot Sauce (p. 93).

Buy Organic/Pastured Chicken, Pork, Lamb & Turkey: These animals have access to the outdoors and eat a more natural diet of organic grains and mixed vegetables, weeds, bugs, and fruit.

Buy Pastured/Grass-Fed Beef & Bison: Cows and bison that live on pastures and eat grass. Pastured, Grass-Fed, and Grass-Finished mean the same thing. These animals are healthier, leaner, have more omega-3s and are sustainably raised.

GMOs: If you're not eating 100% certified organic food, there's an 80 – 90 % chance you're eating (GMOs) genetically modified organisms, which have been linked to negative human and environmental consequences.

Organic Food Recipe

Perfect Hard-Boiled Eggs with Fresh Blueberries

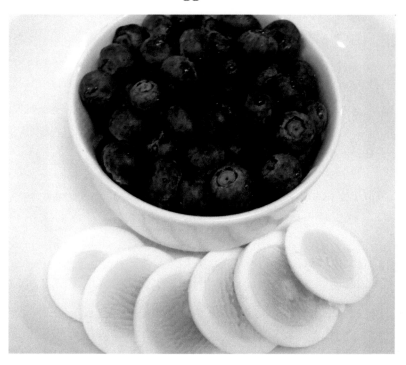

At first glance you may crinkle your noise at this seemingly mismatched breakfast pairing, but wait...

You've heard breakfast is one of the most important meals of the day. Well this twosome gives you what you need.

The eggs provide the protein to build muscle and the berries supply the energy you'll need throughout the day. What you'll also get is protection against cancer, heart disease, diabetes, obesity, and Alzheimer's disease when you choose organic eggs and berries.

The fat and cholesterol in organic eggs is heart-healthy, unlike conventional eggs, and you won't be getting any pesticides served with your organic blueberries.

Tip: Choose breakfast foods for their nutrition & fuel (energy).

Perfect Hard-Boiled Eggs with Fresh Blueberries

Serves 1

What You'll Need

> *eggs, organic, 1 - 2*
>
> *blueberries, organic, fresh, big handful or 1 cup*

To Prepare

The Eggs

1 Place room temperature eggs in a saucepan, cover with cold water, bring to a boil, turn off the heat, cover and let sit for 10 minutes. Place the eggs in an ice water bath for a few minutes to stop them from cooking more. Peel and enjoy. Place extra eggs in the refrigerator with the shells on for up to 6 days.

The Blueberries

1 Wash the berries under cold running water. Eat. Bon Appetit!

Tips

Organic eggs can lower blood cholesterol and protect against cancer and heart disease. Conventional eggs can't. That's because organic eggs have higher levels of omega-3s from a diet rich in vitamins and minerals, instead of GMO corn. So go ahead, enjoy the yolk.

Eggs don't have to be brown to be healthy. The color just indicates the breed of hen. Look for the organic label, or befriend a chicken farmer to ensure you get the healthiest eggs. Pastured chickens lay those golden rich yolks you've seen.

Eat berries in season, June & July in the Northeastern US. They will taste best and be more nutritious. Look online for foods that are in season in your part of the world.

http://www.eatwellguide.org/i.php?pd=Seasonalfoodguides

Rule 4: Choose Fresh Foods

"To be interested in food but not in food production is clearly absurd." - *Wendell Berry*

Squeezing Ripe Melons and Avocados

A friend was having a party and her son requested guacamole. She asked me where to get some. I told her to make it fresh. "No," she said, "Where can I get it, pre-made?" I told her it's easy to make, tastes better than pre-made, and is more nutritious. I also told her she'd have fun making it with her son. She was nervous, but said she'd try it.

One problem; I neglected to tell her how to choose ripe avocados, essential for a creamy end product. They laughed as they attempted to slice through a petrified avocado.

> *Tip: Smell, squeeze, and tap your produce. You'll get to know what's ripe. For avocados choose slightly soft, but not mushy, deep dark green fruits. Follow this link for a guide on picking ripe produce in season.* http://www.eatwellguide.org/i.php?id=Seasonalfoodguides

Eating fresh assures you're eating real food. Fresh can mean; recently picked ripe (most nutrition); in whole form, like a pear; or a combination of fresh foods, like salads. If it's a burger, it was recently ground, as in today. It will most likely not have a wrapper, box or label unless it was freshly frozen, canned, fermented, or baked. Those foods can be healthy too if they contain quality ingredients; think WWOFLES.

What To Look For

The best fresh food is also food that is locally grown. If fresh food isn't local I would question how fresh it is, when it was picked, and how far it has travelled?

> *Fact: Most fresh foods, like vegetables and fruit, lose nutrients within days, often losing as much as 80% of their cancer fighting properties.*

Eat local, ripe, fresh food that's in season as often as you can.

WWOFLES

Fresh Foods

Fresh Foods - Are picked ripe and eaten within hours or days, preferably local, and in-season. Can also be baked (bread), ground (beef), caught (wild fish), frozen fresh (peas), or recently butchered. They're essentially whole foods, packed with their full nutrition and taste. They keep us in touch with the seasons and when purchased locally, support communities.

Examples: Vegetables, Fruit, Bread, Herbs, Meat, Poultry, Fish.

Best Choices: Corn, Lettuce, Greens, Spinach, Avocados, Tomatoes, Grass-Fed Ground Beef, Herbs, Cod, Whole Grain Baguette, Berries.

Recipe Suggestions: Guacamole (next page), Balsamic Dijon Vinaigrette over Greens (p. 67), Garlic Roasted Brussels Sprouts (p. 97), Fish in a Pouch (p. 91).

Note: Choose local, seasonal foods, like fruit and vegetables to guarantee the best flavor, nutrition, and sustainability.

Frozen: Food frozen while fresh can be a healthy alternative to unavailable fresh foods, or out-of-season foods: Fish, Meat, Berries, Corn, Peas, Tomato Sauce, Soup, Bread.

What about Bananas? I prefer not to eat bananas, not because of their sugar content, which I think is a non-issue, but because they have to travel so far, burning up fossil fuel.

Fermentation: Some foods like grapes (wine), cabbages (sauerkraut), and cucumbers (pickles) are fermented while they're fresh, preserving them, and in many cases making them more nutritious. See fermented foods on page 17.

Fresh Food Recipe

Guacamole

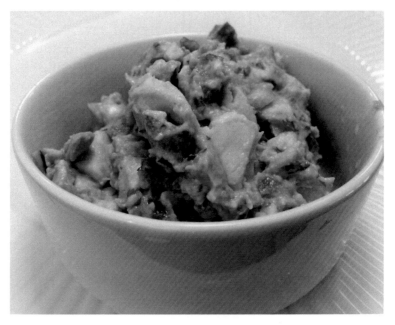

For years I thought eating healthy meant sacrificing great taste, creamy textures, and fun foods. Not so. Learning to prepare fresh, seasonal foods opened up a whole new world for me, leaving behind low-fat, low-carb, and low-taste.

You'll taste fat at its finest, and healthiest, when you bite into this guacamole.

Fresh buying tips

- Shop local and ask your farmer which produce is best
- Look for bright, healthy colors, not necessarily perfect or blemish free
- Greens should be green and crisp, not gray and limp
- Avocados, tomatoes, peaches, plums and other such produce should be firm, yet yield to a gentle squeeze
- Carrots, turnips, beans; should be firm and crack crisply

Guacamole

Serves 4 – 5 (makes about 3 cups)

What you'll need

avocados, 4 ripe, peeled and chopped

tomatoes, plum, 1 large or 2 small , chopped

lime, fresh juice of half or more

red onion, 2- 3 tablespoons or more

jalapeno pepper, 1 tablespoon or more if you like heat, halved, seeded and chopped fine, (you can also use a dash of Tabasco sauce if you prefer)

cilantro, bunch of fresh, chopped (1/2 cup)

sea salt to taste

To Prepare

1 Slice the avocado in half lengthwise by placing it on a cutting board and carefully inserting the knife until you hit the pit. Then rotate the avocado so the knife makes a complete circle, while staying in contact with the pit. Take each half in each palm, and turn each hand counterclockwise, twisting around, and away from each other. Both halves should come apart, with the pit staying in one half. Scoop out the pit with a spoon, or tap with a knife, gently twist, and pop the pit out. Scoop the flesh out with a spoon and place in a bowl.

2 Chop the onion, tomato, pepper, and cilantro. Add them to the bowl with the avocado. Squeeze the lime, add salt and mix to desired consistency. I like mine slightly chunky, but well-blended. Serve with good quality organic tortilla chips, or your favorite vegetables. Bon Appetit!

Tips

Serve immediately for best presentation. Use ripe avocados; slightly soft, but not mushy, deep dark green in color.

Chances are there won't be any leftovers, but in case there are; store in the fridge, covered, with the pit in the bowl.

Rule 5: Choose Local Foods

"Vegetable gardens are more important than houses.... Houses come & go, but soil must be cherished if food is to be grown...."
- Joan Dye Gussow

My Friend The Farmer

Bruce is my friend, however, he's an anomaly. He lives on 8 acres in one of the most congested areas in the United States. What makes him unique is that he is an organic farmer. He owns and runs Old Hook Farm in Emerson, NJ, along with his family.

We visit his farm weekly, buying local produce and gardening supplies, while stepping back in time. My son loves the fresh cherries and cookies on Bruce's shelves, as well as ambling around the farm, climbing on tractors, checking out antiques, and sampling ripe kale, while I chat with Bruce about compost. It's a valuable but vanishing experience.

We know Bruce's family and feel good about supporting his business while he provides my family with nutritious foods, farming knowledge, and enriching experiences. It's a win-win.

Better Health While Supporting Community

Buying locally supports your neighbors and community, and assures you're getting seasonal, fresh food, probably grown without pesticides, picked ripe, nutritionally superior, and sustainable. Local just tastes better!

Get to know your local food providers, whether it's a butcher, fishmonger, farmer or baker. You'll get a better product, personal service, and support a vanishing way of life. When the last local farmer, butcher, and baker shut their businesses, we'll be at the mercy of big conglomerates.

Frequent local farms, farmer's markets, butchers, bakeries, fish markets, join a CSA, and ask your local grocer or healthy supermarket if they can carry local foods.

Get in touch with what you're eating. Overcome squeamishness about where real food comes from, like cow manure. Blindly eating industrially-grown food is unhealthy and unsustainable. Be an activist, eat local and save a farm.

WWOFLES

Local Foods

Local Food - Are seasonal, locally grown, raised, baked, caught, preserved foods. They're typically more nutritious and flavorful, sustainable, minimally processed, and create and support community and social interactions.

Examples: Fruit, Vegetables, Beef, Poultry, Lamb, Game, Dairy, Baked Goods, Fish, Alcohol, Preserves.

*Best Choices***:** Corn, Tomatoes, Spinach, Bread, Cakes, Cheese, Pork, Chicken, Berries, Beef, Lamb, Jams, Jellies, Tomato Sauce.

*Recipe Suggestions***:** Spring Salad With Local Greens, Homemade Croutons & Tahini Dressing (next page), Grilled Green Beans (p. 87), Sautéed Braised Lamb Shanks (p. 103), Acorn Squash Soup (p. 101), Beef Bourguignon a la Jacques Pepin (Beef Stew p. 73), Chicken Fajitas with Homemade Guacamole (p. 83).

Local Raised Animal Products: Cows, Chickens, Pigs, and Lamb. Leaner, more omega-3s, locally, sustainably and humanely raised, access to outdoors, supports your neighbors.

Tip: Befriend your local farmer, butcher, fishmonger, and baker. Ask them what's fresh, what they eat, and how they prepare their food.

Start a Garden: Elliot Coleman is an excellent organic gardening resource. http://www.fourseasonfarm.com

Want to read more about eating local? Read, *This Organic Life: Confessions of a Suburban Homesteader*, by Joan Dye Gussow.

Local Food Recipe

Spring Salad With Local Greens, Homemade Croutons & Tahini Dressing

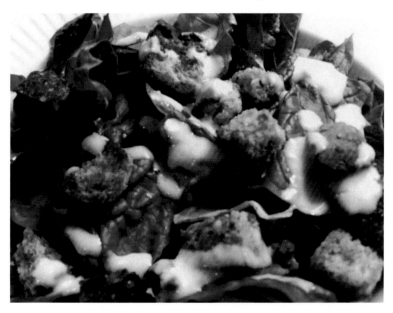

Growing up, my Greek mother couldn't get me to eat a green salad. Meat and potatoes were my thing. Thankfully, I've changed. I still love meat, but I've learned to appreciate local, seasonal fruit and vegetables. Maybe it's because my palate grew up, or because I grow organic vegetables. The tastiest, healthiest vegetables are the ones that are local, in-season, and picked ripe.

You'll love this fresh, crisp, and fast salad made with homemade croutons and creamy, lemony tahini sauce. Go to your local farmer's market or farm to get the spinach, your local baker for a fresh baguette, and an ethnic market for tahini. Make shopping for food an adventure.

Spring Salad With Local Greens, Homemade Croutons & Tahini Dressing

Serves 3-4

What You'll Need

greens- kale, spinach, Boston & romaine lettuce, arugula,

or your favorite in-season greens, 3 large handfuls

red onion, 1/4 medium onion, chopped

sea salt and pepper to taste

Croutons: Recipe Below

day old bread, couple of slices, cubed

olive oil, extra virgin, couple of tablespoons

sea salt to taste

Tahini Dressing: Recipe Below

tahini, 1 tablespoon

garlic, 1 clove, crushed or finely chopped

lemon, juice of half or more

water, 2-3 tablespoons

sea salt, pinch

To Prepare

Croutons - Preheat oven to 350 degrees. Cube your favorite bread, place on baking sheet, drizzle with olive oil, salt and toss. Bake till crispy golden, for 3 – 5 minutes, or until golden brown. Check often as they burn quickly. Remove and let cool.

Tahini Dressing - Combine tahini, garlic, lemon juice, water, and salt, blend well.

Salad – Wash and coarsely chop greens to bite size pieces and place in bowl. Toss in croutons and drizzle with tahini. Bon Appetit!

Rule 6: Choose Ethnic (Traditional) Foods

"The best way to execute French cooking is to get good and loaded and whack the hell out of a chicken."
- Julia Child

Greek Immigrants and Feta Cheese

In 1969 my parents stepped off a boat in NYC. Fresh from Greece, via Australia, they quickly assimilated into the American way of life. Soon divorced, my mom raised three kids on Big Macs and Ding Dongs due to economic necessity and ignorance, intermixed with traditional Greek staples like Feta cheese, olive oil and dandelion greens.

As I matured and started a family, I became proud of my ethnic heritage, and left behind my fast food upbringing. I'm pleased at the fact that my 14-year-old daughter loves Greek food and has never eaten in a fast food chain. My friends think I'm depriving her, but I joke and say, Anna's never had a McDonald's Happy Meal and yet, remarkably, she's happy. They don't always get the joke.

Ethnic Can Mean Quality Food

Today, when I want quality food for my family, I buy traditional Greek foods like olives, extra virgin olive oil, and goat's milk feta cheese, which my family has eaten for centuries. When we go back 4-5 generations to our ancestors we'll find some of the healthiest foods available; whole, fresh, local, seasonal foods served in traditional ways, and centered around social customs that enrich our lives, as well as our health.

Recently I visited an Italian client's home to ask her husband his secrets about growing tomatoes. I was offered lunch, politely declined, then found myself sitting in front of a six-course meal.

I enjoyed salad from the their garden, homemade bread, fresh roasted peppers & mozzarella cheese, a nectarine, apricot and homemade wine. I was sent home with 3 gallons of wine and two jars of tomato sauce, canned fresh from the garden.

In my opinion, this tradition of food preparation and hospitality is too seldom experienced today. We would do right by our children to turn off all of our electronic devices and make sauce together. Eat Ethnic.

Whole, Wild, Organic, Fresh, Local, Ethnic, Seasonal

WWOFLES

Ethnic Foods
(Traditional)

Ethnic (Traditional) - Foods prepared and eaten according to cultural, social, national, regional or religious traditions that sustain health and provide communal benefits.

Examples: Greek, Italian, Thai, Mexican, Spanish, Chinese, Jewish, Indian, French, & Cuisines - Mediterranean, Asian, Middle Eastern, etc...

Best Choices: Chick Peas, Avocados, Sesame Seeds, Tomatoes, Cheese, Collard Greens, Dandelion Greens, Olive oil, Olives, Peppers, Coconut Milk, Garlic, Soy Sauce, Cayenne Pepper, Curry, Wine, French Baguette, and herbs and spices such as - Turmeric, Cinnamon, Oregano, Basil, Ginger, Thyme, Cumin.

Recipe Suggestions: Edamame Hummus (next page) Greek Village (Horiatiki) Salad (p. 55), Guacamole (p. 37), Horseradish Hummus (p. 65), Mu Shu Chicken with Lettuce Wraps p. (71), Beef Bourguignon a la Jacques Pepin (French Beef Stew) (p. 73), Nicoise Salad with Tuna and Spring Veggies (p. 79), Gourmet French Veggies (p. 19).

*Ethnic meals have traditionally depended on local, seasonal, fresh, whole foods, prepared in simple ways that maximize taste and create communal experiences, which are, unfortunately, missing from many of our dining room tables.

Note: I know I told you to buy local a couple pages back, but sometimes you want ethnic foods that are not produced locally, like olive oil. The choice is yours to make.

Ethnic Food Recipe

Edamame Hummus

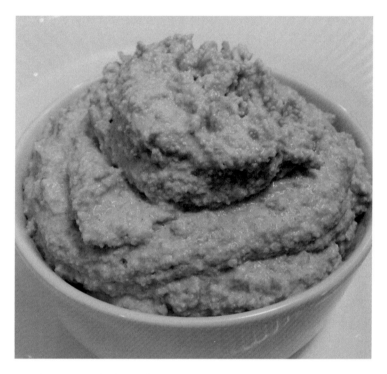

This is probably the tastiest hummus I've ever had. Rich and creamy, with a beautiful earth green color, I swear I taste a hint of Parmesan cheese, but it can't be because this dish is dairy-free.

Get out your food processor, set aside 5 minutes, and create this healthy, delicious treat!

Tip: Organic edamame beans (soy beans) are a great vegetable source of a complete protein and a healthier form of soy than the stuff we get in processed GMO foods like bread, cakes, & cookies.

The healthiest soy products are fermented: Like Miso, Tamari, and Tempeh. Make sure they are organic or they're 90% likely to contain GMOs.

Edamame Hummus

Serves 4-5

What You'll Need

edamame beans, 1 cup, cooked, fresh or frozen (defrosted)

tahini, 1 tablespoon or more

lemon juice, 2 tablespoons, or more

garlic, 1-2 cloves, crushed

olive oil, extra virgin, 2 tablespoon or more, depending on the thickness you like

sea salt to taste

To Prepare

1 Combine beans, tahini, lemon juice, and garlic in food processor. Process while drizzling olive oil through feed tube. Continuing to process until you've achieved a smooth consistency.

2 Season with salt to taste, process briefly, and serve with a final drizzle of olive oil.

Serving Suggestions

Serve with organic tortilla chips; whole grain or rice crackers; or fresh seasonal veggies.

Ethnic Tip

Find out what your great grandparents ate. How did they prepare their food? What did they eat at certain times of the year? There's a good chance their food practices would benefit you today.

Use fresh lemons and limes in recipes. Bottled lemon and lime juice doesn't taste as good and contains preservatives.

Rule 7: Choose Seasonal Foods

"Let things taste of what they are."
- Alice Waters

Tasteless Tomatoes

I went to Greece for my honeymoon and fell in love with Greek village salads (recipe follows).

I loved them so much I decided to make them a year-round staple. Novice mistake. I soon realized that the salads tasted mysteriously better in summer, even though I used the same ingredients year round. Why?

I live in New Jersey, famous for tomatoes, the kind that come to mind when you think of food perfection - big, juicy, red, sweet. I wasn't aware back then that they're only in season from July to September.

I'd go to the supermarket in January and buy what looked like a tomato. What I got was a tasteless, nutritionally deficient object; red and shiny like a tomato, but not the real thing at all. I wouldn't think of buying a tomato in January anymore. Parents, take note if you're kids won't eat their veggies: Foods eaten out of season don't taste nearly as good as in-season foods, especially vegetables.

Break The "What's for Dinner" Monotony

Many of us get stuck in a rut of eating the same ol' foods, healthy or otherwise. We get fed up and declare, "Enough, I'm getting that crumb bun I've been eyeing."

Seasonal eating gives you more options so you don't have to rebel. Studies show they have superior nutrition, taste better, offer variety, and put you in rhythm with the earth.

This last point helps you eat healthier. Following the seasons and eating natural foods in your part of the world helps you eat more whole foods, picked ripe (most tasty and nutritious), and locally grown (sustainable and supports your community).

Each season means new foods to try, the return of favorite recipes shared with family and friends, and a break in the monotony that life can become. Eat the seasons.

Whole, Wild, Organic, Fresh, Local, Ethnic, Seasonal

WWOFLES

← →

Seasonal Foods

Seasonal Foods – Grown & harvested during the current season, excel in nutrition and flavor, are typically less expensive, support local business, offer variety, decrease pollution & greenhouse emissions, and connect us to the earth.

Spring: Spinach, Kale, Arugula, Carrots, Asparagus, Artichokes, Dandelion Greens, New Potatoes, Lamb, Crab, Sardines, Scallops.

Summer: Tomatoes, Cucumbers, Zucchini, Beets, Eggplant, Squash, Green Beans, Peas, Peaches, Berries, Plums, Cherries, Melons, Pickles, Haddock, Salmon, Lobster, Parsley, Basil, Oregano, Cilantro, Mint.

Fall: Apples, Pears, Cabbage, Cauliflower, Brussels Sprouts, Cranberries, Butternut Squash, Pumpkin, Sweet Potatoes, Mushrooms, Grapes, Oregano, Thyme, Duck, Pork.

Winter: Kale, Broccoli, Collards, Spinach, Escarole, Carrots, Oranges, Grapefruit, Sage, Rosemary, Beef.

Tip: Give kids seasonal fruit and veggies. They taste better! Put them out in ripening bowls on the counter and watch them go. Eat canned and preserved foods throughout the year that were preserved when they were ripe and in-season (e.g., blueberry jam, pickles, sauerkraut, tomato sauce).

Seasonal Recipes

Winter pp. 65 - 73
Spring pp. 75 - 83
Summer pp. 85 - 93
Fall pp. 95 - 103

Seasonal Food Recipe

Greek Village (Horiatiki) Salad

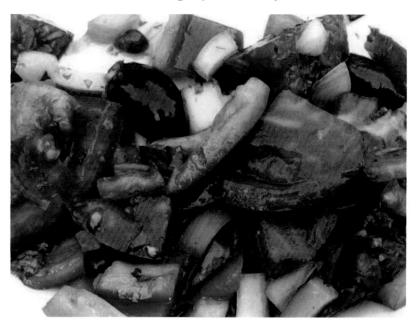

If you know any Greeks, you're probably aware they're passionate about their salads, made with the freshest ingredients, prepared in the simplest way. The salad below is one of the countless variations of a Horiatiki, pronounced, "hor-ya-ti-ki", which means village.

Using seasonal foods to make your salads and other dishes allows you to elevate a seemingly mundane health staple into an up-lifting dining experience, full of memories of seasons past.

*"To every thing there is a season, and a time to every purpose...
A time to be born, and a time to die; a time to plant, and a time
to pluck that which is planted." - The Bible*

Greek Village (Horiatiki) Salad

Serves 4-5

What you'll need

beefsteak tomatoes, (or your favorite), 2 large, cut in ½ inch chunks

cucumber, ½ of whole or 1 cup, chopped into ½inch pieces

green pepper, ½, chopped into ½ inch pieces

kalamata olives, handful, pitted or not

capers, 1 tablespoon with some juice drizzled in

feta cheese, 1 ounce good quality, made from goat or sheep's milk, crumbled

Dressing

red onion, ¼ of whole, chopped fine

olive oil, extra virgin (preferably from Greece), 2 tablespoons or more

red wine vinegar, 2 teaspoons or more

lemon, a big squeeze

oregano, thyme, parsley, dill, start with 1 tablespoon of each fresh or 1 teaspoon dried

sea salt & pepper to taste

variations: lettuce, grilled veggies, roasted peppers, caramelized onions, flank steak, or whatever you love

To Prepare

1 Place all salad ingredients in a large bowl and add dressing. Squeeze the lemon over the salad, add the cheese or let everyone do it them selves, and serve. That's it! Bon Appetit!

Pantry, Prep, & Cooking Tips

Pantry, Prep, & Cooking Tips

1 Let meat come to room temperature before cooking.

2 Dry meat before cooking, and don't crowd the meat when trying to grill, sear, or brown. Otherwise the meat will steam.

3 Measure, chop and prep all ingredients before cooking,

4 Cut extra ingredients and store in containers in the fridge. On Sunday, wash all your greens, cut & bag them for the week.

5 Generally, roast meats at low oven temperatures (250 – 300 degrees F) for 2 – 6 hours for maximum tenderness.

6 Generally, roast vegetables like potatoes and broccoli at high oven temperatures (375 – 425 degrees F).

7 Herbs – ratio of fresh herbs to dried is 3 to 1. For example 1 tablespoon of fresh oregano would = 1 teaspoon of dried.

8 Try to use fresh, in-season herbs to improve flavors. Store fresh herbs in vase with water or in the fridge.

9 Use extra virgin, cold pressed olive oil as your primary fat source for flavor and nutrition. Cooking dulls the flavor of olive oil, so reserve some for drizzling over your finished dishes.

10 Use a good quality balsamic vinegar. How do you know? Look for "traditional" on the label, with only 1 ingredient – grapes. It will be thick, syrupy and sweet. Avoid added sugars.

11 Always use a sharp knife.

12 Cook with the wine you like to drink.

13 Clean up as you go.

14 Which potatoes to use?

> Baking potatoes: course skin - Russets or Idaho, good for baking, mashing and frying.

> Boiling potatoes: waxy skin – Red, Gold, Yellow. Good for soups, casseroles, potato salad, roasting, and barbecuing.

15 For the best roasted potatoes, boil waxy potatoes in chicken or veggie stock until done, drain, toss with olive oil, season and roast on 400 degrees F till colored and crispy.

16 Choose recipes and meals with foods that are in season.

17 Puree vegetable soups for creaminess without the cream.

18 Serve and keep food warm for best flavor.

19 Use the freshest, best ingredients you can find. Your food will taste better, guaranteed.

20 Salt – I use sea salt, freshly ground, for most dishes, except when grilling or making a rib roast, when I use kosher salt. Kosher salt is more course than table salt. I don't use table salt because it may not be pure salt.

21 Use natural sweeteners like honey, agave, or pure cane sugar. Avoid artificial sweeteners. Try cinnamon as a no-calorie sweetener.

22 Mustard: I recommend authentic Dijon, French and grainy stone ground with no additives or preservatives.

23 Typically, I use red onions for salads & dressings, yellow onions for cooking, and Vidalia or Spanish onions for grilling.

24 Cook pasta al dente; which means toothy, not mushy. The sugars dissolve slower in your body keeping blood sugar steady.

25 Gently fry eggs on low heat in olive oil for soft, tender whites.

Seasonal Recipes

Winter

Spring

Summer

Fall

Seasonal Recipes

Winter

Spring

Summer

Fall

Winter Recipes

Horseradish Hummus

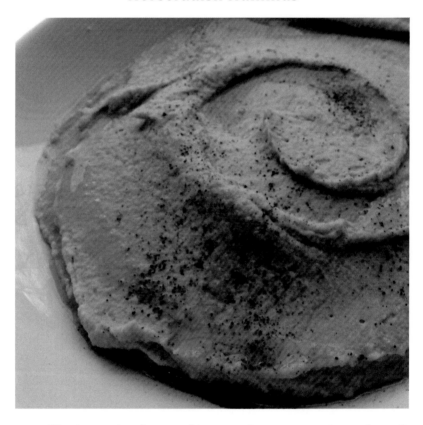

Hummus is the perfect snack, or appetizer, for after school, pre–dinner, or during parties. This is a classic recipe with some horseradish sauce thrown in for zing.

Preparation tips

When using canned beans, I like to use a fork to lift the beans out of the can over the food processor bowl. This brings some of the liquid in which I think adds to the flavor and creates the perfect consistency

Be creative, add: roasted red peppers, olives, edamame, hot peppers, chilies, cilantro.

Horseradish Hummus

Serves 4-5

What you'll need

garbanzo beans, 2 cups, cooked, (or 15 oz can)

tahini, 1 tablespoon

lemon, juice of ½ or whole to taste

garlic cloves, 1-2, peeled and crushed

olive oil, extra virgin, 2 tablespoon or more, depending on thickness you like

prepared horseradish, start with 2 teaspoons

sea salt to taste

pinch of paprika for garnish

To prepare

1 Combine beans, tahini, lemon juice, horseradish, and garlic in food processor. Process while drizzling olive oil through feed tube. Continuing to process until you've achieved a smooth consistency.

2 Season with salt to taste, process briefly, and serve with a final drizzle of olive oil. Bon Appetit!

Garlic tip

Use a garlic press to crush your garlic. Many chefs believe it gives your dishes more flavor, and I agree, especially when using it raw.

Serving suggestion

Present with a vegetable crudité, whole grain pita, or crackers.

Winter Recipes
Balsamic Dijon Vinaigrette Dressing

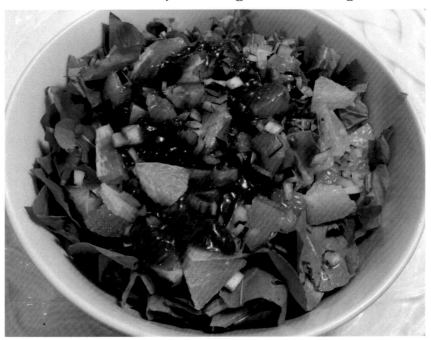

This may seem obvious, but the secret of great balsamic vinegar dressings is to use the best quality balsamic vinegar you can find. It will cost you a bit more, but it's worth it for the flavor.

The best quality balsamic vinegar will be thick, syrupy, sweet, and have a tart tang to it. It may have the word, "traditional", or "traditionale" on the label, it comes from Modena Italy, and will generally be sold in gourmet food stores. I occasionally find some in discount department stores.

Beware of cheap imitations with artificial ingredients and added refined sugars. The words "balsamic glaze" are a dead giveaway. The one and only ingredient should be grapes.

I also recommend you use a good quality Dijon mustard made with white wine.

Balsamic Dijon Vinaigrette Dressing

Serves 4-5

What you'll need

Dressing

olive oil, extra virgin, 1 tablespoon

balsamic vinegar, 2 tablespoons, very good quality

Dijon mustard, 2 tablespoons

red onion, 1/4 of a medium, or 3 tablespoons chopped

sea salt & pepper, to taste

Salad Options: Use winter greens

arugula, or kale romaine, chard, dandelion greens

clementine, or your favorite citrus fruit, peeled and sliced into small sections

sunflower seeds, toasted

To prepare

1 Wash and chop greens, and place in a large bowl. Top greens with clementine's and sunflower seeds.

2 In a small bowl mix together the vinegar, mustard and onions. Slowly pour in oil while whisking to create an emulsion (thick liquid). Season with salt, drizzle over salad and gently toss. Bon Appetit!

Toasting Sunflower Seeds: Spread on a baking sheet, sprinkle with salt and place in a 350 oven. Cook for 3-5 minutes, checking every minute and giving them a quick shake to move them around. Make sure they don't burn. Remove when they look toasted, brownish.

Winter Recipes

Kale Soup with San Marzano Tomatoes

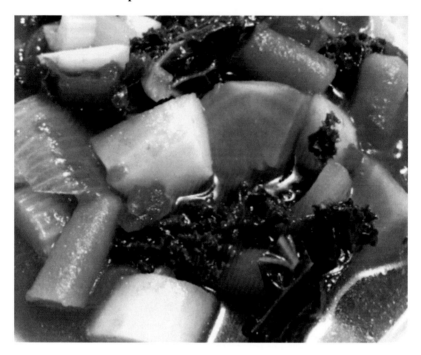

Liven up traditional vegetable soup with some hearty kale and sweet San Marzano tomatoes grown in the soil of Mt. Vesuvius in Italy. This soup was a big hit at my house on a cold Sunday afternoon.

Soup is a great low-calorie food that when it's vegetable based, provides good nutrition, and will keep you full longer. As always, buy organic when possible. I served this with sautéed wild sole in white wine and lemon.

San Marzano Tomatoes – These tomatoes are grown in the volcanic soil near Mt Vesuvius in Italy, which is supposed to contribute to their umami (the 5th taste). They will transcend any dish in which they are added into a sublime chef-d'oeuvre. Look for them canned with an official DOP seal on the label. You can also grow them from seeds in your garden.

Kale Soup with San Marzano Tomatoes

Serves 7-10 (freeze the leftovers)

What you'll need

vegetable or chicken stock, 4 cups, low sodium

kale, Dinosaur, Laminator, or Tuscan, 2 large handfuls, chopped

carrots, 3 large, peeled and cubed

parsnips, 3 large, peeled and cubed

sweet potatoes, 1 large, peeled and cubed

onion, 1 large, chopped

San Marzano canned tomatoes, 16 oz.

thyme, 3 tablespoons fresh chopped, or 1 teaspoon dried

bay leaves, 3 dried

sea salt & pepper to taste

To prepare

1 Add all ingredients to a heavy Dutch oven or stock pot, season to taste, and bring to a boil. Immediately reduce to a simmer and cook for 30 minutes.

2 After 30 minutes add kale and cook until vegetables are al dente - about 30 minutes. Do not overcook vegetables.

Tips

Authentic San Marzano Tomatoes will have an official seal on the can. They have a distinct sweet flavor to them.

When buying or making soup, consider tomato or vegetable based instead of heavy cream-based soups. Some thick soups are just pureed vegetables like butternut squash or carrot soup, without the addition of heavy cream or butter.

Winter Recipes

Mu Shu Chicken

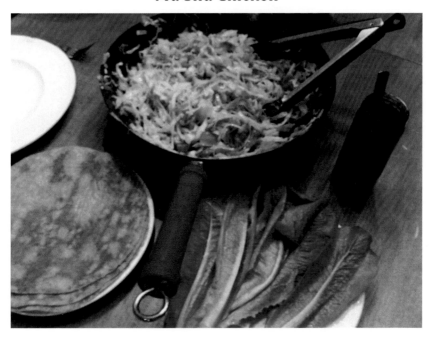

My family likes take-out Chinese food once in a while. But we also like to know what's in our food, so we make this dish at home and leave out the egg. (my son is allergic) and sugar (it doesn't need it). You can substitute beef or shrimp, or make it vegan by leaving out the meat or fish.

Preparation tips

Slice the cabbage and chicken into thin strips. Crush, or finely grate the garlic and ginger for more flavor. You can peel the carrots into strips with a peeler, instead of julienning, which takes some knife skill. Cook until the cabbage is tender, but al dente. You don't want mush. Season at the end, so you don't add too much soy sauce. The wok gets crowded, so buy or use the biggest one you can find, and use tongs to mix.

Mu Shu Chicken

Serves 5

What you'll need

chicken, 1 lb boneless, skinless, chicken thighs, sliced thin

onion, 1 medium, yellow, sliced thin

green cabbage, 1 medium head, finely shredded, or sliced thin

carrots, 3 medium, julienned, or peeled into strips

ginger, fresh, 2 tablespoons peeled and minced or finely grated,

garlic, crushed or finely grated, 1 tablespoon or 1 large clove

hoisin sauce, 3 tablespoons, plus more for serving

low-sodium soy sauce, 3 tablespoons or to taste

sesame oil, 2 tablespoons

olive oil, extra virgin, 3 tablespoons

sea salt & black pepper to taste

romaine lettuce leaves or flour tortillas for wrapping

How to prepare

1 Combine 1 tablespoon hoisin and soy sauce, the sesame oil, 1/2 the garlic and 1/2 the ginger, salt, pepper, and add to the sliced chicken in a mixing bowl. Toss to coat evenly. Marinate the chicken, covered, at room temperature for 10 to 20 minutes.

2 When done marinating, heat a large wok or skillet over high heat with 2 tablespoons of the oil. When the wok is hot, spoon in the chicken and stir often until browned and almost cooked through, about 3-5 minutes. Remove the chicken to a plate.

3 Add another tablespoon of oil and stir fry the remaining garlic and ginger for 1 minute, stirring often. Then add the onion slices, and cook, stirring often, for 2 more minutes. Next, add the cabbage and carrots and cook, stirring often, until just browned and almost al dente (tender but not mushy), about 2-4 minutes.

4 Add the chicken back in with the juices from the plate. Stir fry for 2 minutes until the chicken is done, then add the remaining soy sauce and hoisin and adjust to taste. Serve immediately with tortillas, or lettuce leaves and hoisin sauce, or serve over rice. Bon Appetit!

Winter Recipes

Jacques Pepin's Beef Bourguignon
(French Beef Stew in Red Wine)

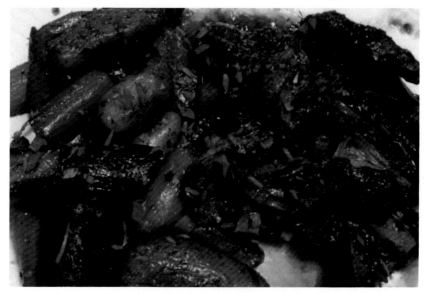

Adapted from Jacques Pepin in *Food & Wine*.

Melt in your mouth unctuousness is the best way to describe this dish. Perfect for a lazy autumn or winter Sunday afternoon, or anytime you want stick to your ribs goodness.

I thought that the liquid in a stew was always water or some type of stock, like veggie, beef or chicken. When I watched Jacques Pepin make this stew on PBS by pouring in an entire bottle of red wine, and no other liquid, that got my attention.

I modified this dish by using a lower cooking temperature, and added a can of San Marzano tomatoes, for color and taste. I typically serve this dish over French style gourmet vegetables p. 21, or you can ladle over pasta, rice, or any vegetables or grains you like.

Jacques Pepin's Beef Bourguignon

Serves 5-6 with leftovers, 4-6 hours cooking time

What you'll need

beef chuck, 2 pounds, cut into 1 inch cubes (local, grass fed)

short ribs, 4 large, on the bone (local, grass fed)

bacon, 2 thick slices, smoked, nitrate free, chopped

red wine, 1 bottle of your favorite, I like a Bordeaux or Burgundy

carrots, 3 large, chopped fine

onion, 1 large, chopped fine

celery, 3 stalks, chopped fine

garlic, 5 cloves, chopped fine

olive oil, extra virgin, 4-5 tablespoon

San Marzano tomatoes, one 28 ounce can

thyme, fresh, 2 tablespoons,, or 1 tablespoon dried, chopped

bay leaves, 3 dried

sea salt & pepper to taste

To Prepare

1 Preheat the oven to 250°. Heat over medium-high heat a large enameled cast-iron casserole or Dutch oven. Arrange the meat in a single layer and cook, turning once browned, on all sides. Do not crowd the meat. Remove to a plate and repeat with any remaining meat.

2 Adjust the heat to medium, add the bacon and cook until crispy, stirring often. Add the chopped onion and 1 tablespoon olive oil and cook over low-medium heat, stirring occasionally until the onion is softened, 5 minutes, scraping up the bits of meat. Add the garlic, carrots, and celery, and cook for 5 more minutes. Add enough wine to scrape the remaining bits of meat from the bottom. Add the rest of the wine, bay leaves and thyme, season with salt and pepper and bring to a boil.

3 Cover the casserole and transfer it to the oven. Cook the stew for 4-6 hours, until the meat is very tender and the sauce is flavorful. (It will probably be ready in 1 1/2 hours, but cooking it for 4-6 hours transforms it from a good dish to a masterpiece.) To serve, ladle over vegetables, noodles or pasta, like orzo, and garnish with fresh chopped parsley and drizzle of olive oil. Bon Appetit!

Spring Recipes

Garlic, Lime, Cilantro Dressing

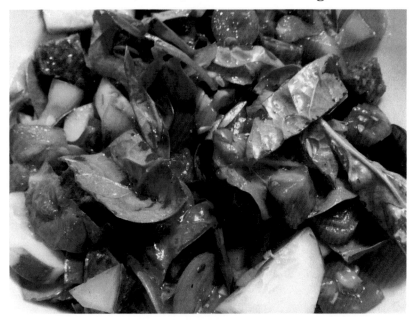

Do you get bored of the same ol' salad dressing? Me too! That's why I mix things up with flavorful seasonal dressings.

As a rule I don't use bottled dressing because they're typically inferior quality, full of artificial ingredients and refined sugars, and they're so easy to make at home that buying processed salad dressing doesn't make sense to me. Just remember to use the freshest, best quality, and seasonal ingredients when possible.

The secret of this dressing is the fresh cilantro, good quality extra virgin olive oil and ripe limes. You can adjust the amounts of each ingredient to your liking.

Nutritional Benefits

The garlic, lime, cilantro and olive oil have anti-inflammatory and anti-oxidant properties that fight disease. They also taste great.

74

Garlic, Lime, Cilantro Dressing

Serves 4 - 5

What you'll need

lime, fresh juice of 1 (about 2 tablespoons)

olive oil, extra virgin, 2 tablespoons,

garlic, 1 clove, crushed or finely chopped

cilantro, fresh, 1 handful, chopped

honey, 1 tablespoon

sea salt & pepper to taste

To prepare

1 Add all ingredients to a bowl, except the olive oil, and mix together.

2 Slowly add the oil while whisking to make an emulsion (thick liquid). Salt and pepper to taste. Serve over your favorite salad or use as a dip for veggies or chips. Bon Appetit!

Salad tips

You can use any spring mix, spinach, arugula, kale, or your favorite lettuce. You can also add your favorite ingredients including red onions, roasted peppers, olives, croutons, or a protein like chicken, fish, beans, or cheese.

People either love or hate Cilantro, there's no in-between. Some scientists say it has to do with taste buds. If you're a cilantro lover, choose the brightest green stems you can find or grown them in your garden or sunny windowsill.

Don't add the dressing until you're ready to serve. I always make extra salad and let everyone pour the dressing onto their own plates so my leftovers aren't soggy the next day.

Spring Recipes

Wild Salmon over Spinach

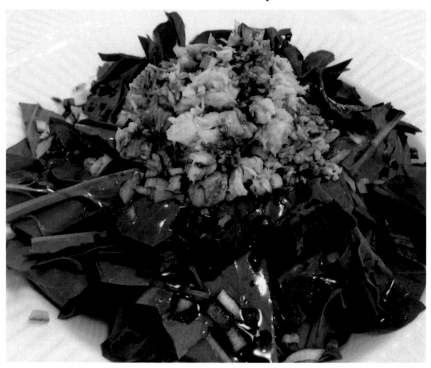

I often make this salad for lunch, and every time I do I can't believe how simple it is and how good it tastes! It only takes a couple of ingredients and you have a healthy salad in 5 minutes!

Canned wild salmon is a cheaper and easier way to get the health benefits of omega 3's.

Other quick & delicious snack/meal ideas

- Smoked sardines with balsamic vinegar and whole grain crackers
- Cheese, tomatoes, olives, olive oil, & good crusty bread
- Hummus with seasonal veggies
- Whole grain sourdough bread with homemade jams

Wild Salmon over Spinach

Serves 1-2

What you'll need

wild salmon, one 3 ounce can

spinach or lettuce, 2 cups or 1 large bunch

red onion, 1 tablespoon, chopped

grape tomatoes, 5, sliced in half

olive oil, extra virgin, a drizzle

balsamic vinegar, a drizzle

sea salt, pinch, and freshly ground black pepper

To Prepare

1 Wash and dry spinach. Chop, place in bowl.

2 Finely chop red onion, halve tomatoes, and place over spinach.

3 Open can of salmon, drain, and flake with a fork over salad.

4 Drizzle olive oil and vinegar, season with salt and pepper. Bon Appetit!

Delicious secrets

You've heard this before, if you want the best tasting, most satisfying foods, start with excellent ingredients, especially with simple dishes like this one. I use the best quality olive oil and balsamic vinegar I can afford, and insist on crisp, in-season greens. I'm convinced that's why my kids will try, and enjoy many foods that other kids won't.

Summer Recipes

Nicoise Salad with Tuna and Spring Veggies

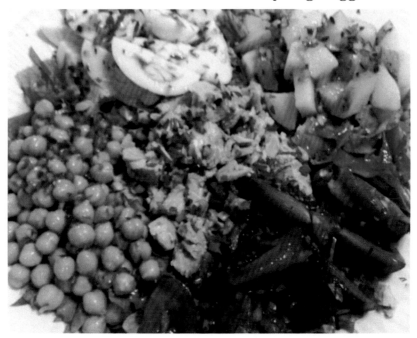

I often hear people complain about eating the same ol' salad, with the same ol' dressing, yet again. I tell them to try a Nicoise style salad, classically French and traditionally composed of tomatoes, green beans, tuna, hard-boiled eggs, Nicoise olives, anchovies, and dressed with a vinaigrette, with or without a bed of lettuce. It has many variations making it perfect when you're in the mood for something different.

This is one of my favorite versions using new potatoes, garbanzo beans, and heirloom tomatoes (I grow Purple Cherokees in my garden). You can also try artichoke hearts, roasted peppers, and cheese. Use what's seasonal.

Tip: Serve this dish with the potatoes and eggs just warm.

Nicoise Salad with Tuna and Spring Veggies

Serves 4-5

What you'll need

> tuna, canned, 3-6 ounce
>
> salad greens, 3 - 6 cups (2 large romaine heads) or your favorite greens, like kale or spinach
>
> nicoise olives, or your favorite
>
> garbanzo beans, 1 cup, canned, drained
>
> tomatoes, 2 medium, halved and quartered (use your favorite in-season)
>
> roasted red peppers, 1 large, chopped
>
> eggs, hard boiled, 4
>
> new potatoes, 5 small, boiled, diced
>
> ### Dressing
>
> shallots or red onion, 2 tablespoons, chopped fine
>
> olive oil, extra virgin, 1/4 cup
>
> red wine vinegar, 1/3 cup
>
> Dijon mustard, 1 tablespoon
>
> sea salt & pepper to taste

To Prepare

1 To make the dressing, chop onions fine, place them with the vinegar and mustard in a small bowl. Slowly drizzle in olive oil while whisking vigorously until all oil is used and you create an emulsion (all ingredients combine and thicken). Season with salt and pepper, set aside.

2 Wash, cube, and boil potatoes until tender, 8-10 minutes, strain and set aside.

3 Place eggs in saucepan, cover with tap water, bring to a boil, turn off the heat, cover, and let sit for 10 minutes. Then rinse under cold water, peel, cut into quarters, set aside.

4 Cut peppers into a rough chop. Open and drain beans. Wash and coarsely chop the salad greens.

5 Spread out the greens on a large dish. Place the tuna at the center, and the potatoes, tomatoes, beans, and eggs around the perimeters. Drizzle with the salad dressing and serve. Bon Appetit!

Spring Recipes
BBQ Sauce Burgers

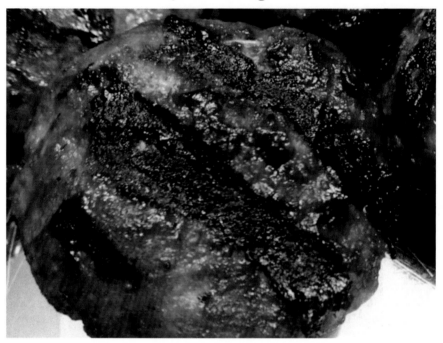

    I believe burgers can be healthy as well as delicious.
The way to guarantee that is to buy grass-fed beef or bison. In addition to being full of flavor, the meat is higher in omega-3s, have less saturated fat, and the animals are sustainably raised.

    I also like to mix it up with organic ground chicken or turkey. I recommend a mix of white and dark meat, or just dark meat; otherwise the burger is too dry in my opinion.

    Sometimes, when dining out, you'll see grass fed or organic burgers on the menu. I recommend ordering them.

    This recipe was inspired by a trip to the grocery store where I saw pre-made BBQ turkey burgers in the butcher's case. It's a nice change up once in a while.

BBQ Sauce Burgers

Serves 4, (makes four, 4 ounce burgers)

What you'll need

grass-fed ground beef, turkey, or chicken, 1 pound

Breadcrumbs, whole wheat, 1/4 cup

your favorite BBQ sauce, 3 tbsp. plus more to baste Burgers

onion, 1 small, chopped fine

sea salt & pepper to taste

To prepare

1 Preheat grill to medium/high heat.

2 Mix the ground meat with all of the ingredients and form into patties.

3 Place on hot grill for 5 minutes, then turn over. Brush with barbecue sauce, let cook for 5 minutes more then turn over again. Baste burgers again, let cook for another 5 minutes and remove from heat and serve.

Cooking temps

Beef - 135 degrees F for medium rare (recommended)

Chicken & Turkey - 160 degrees F

Tip – Take meat off the grill 10 degrees below desired doneness. It will continue to cook about 10 degrees.

Serving suggestion

Do the bun thing or simply serve over a bed of greens with diced red pickled onion, cucumber pickles, or caramelized onions.

Spring Recipes

Chicken Fajitas with Homemade Guacamole

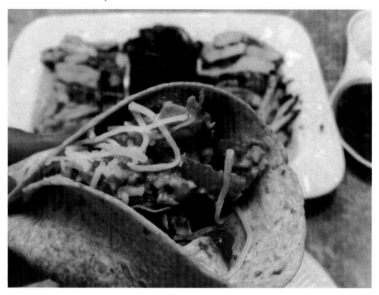

These fajitas offer something that everyone can enjoy and agree on- variety. Serve them with multiple ingredient options that they pick themselves to make their own creations:

- chicken, beef, or shrimp
- tomatoes
- cheese
- guacamole
- salsa
- peppers
- onions
- broccoli
- lettuce

Place all the ingredients in bowls on the table and let them have a go at them.

Chicken Fajitas with Homemade Guacamole

Serves 3-5

What you'll need

Fajitas

whole wheat tortillas, or lettuce for wraps

chicken breasts, 5, skinless, boneless

red pepper, 1

red onion, 1

broccoli, 1 stalk of florets

salsa, one 8 ounce jar

Mexican cheese blend, grated (many stores will carry this)

fajita seasoning

olive oil

Guacamole

avocados, 4 ripe, peeled and chopped

tomatoes, plum, 1 large or 2 small , chopped

lime, fresh juice of half or more

red onion, 2- 3 tablespoons or more

jalapeno pepper, 1 tablespoon or more if you like heat, halved, seeded and chopped fine, (you can also use a dash of Tabasco sauce if you prefer)

cilantro, bunch of fresh, chopped (1/2 cup)

sea salt to taste

To Prepare - Fajita recipe

1 Marinate chicken breasts in olive oil, lime, chopped cilantro, fajita seasoning salt & pepper.

2 Chop onions, peppers and broccoli and sauté in olive oil for 10 minutes over medium heat and set aside.

3 Grill or sauté chicken and slice in long strips. Heat tortillas in aluminum foil on grill or in oven. Place ingredients in serving bowls and have everyone assemble their favorite ingredients.

Guacamole Recipe

1 Peel and coarsely chop the avocados. Chop onion & tomato. Mix the avocados, onion, tomato, chopped cilantro, squeeze of lime and salt together and serve with other condiments. Bon Appetit!

Summer Recipes

Bean, Corn, & Avocado Salad

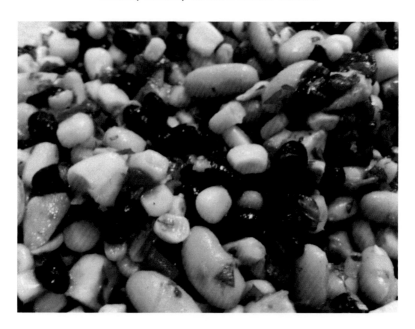

This dish is a fast and easy staple in my house, full of plant protein, fiber and flavor. A perfect side dish to any grilled meats, or as a main course served with soup.

Sometimes I forget about the canned beans in the cupboard and this recipe is a perfect reminder of how good and easy it can be to use them. If you're a good planner, I recommend buying dried beans and soaking them overnight for even more flavor. If I can't get local fresh corn, I'll use frozen organic.

Pantry tips

Always have assorted cans of organic canned beans on hand for salads, soups and dips like hummus: Black, kidney, garbanzo (chick peas), cannellini, etc.

Keep frozen organic corn and peas in the freezer for when you can't get fresh, or when they're not in season.

Bean, Corn, & Avocado Salad

Serves 3-5 with leftovers

What you'll need

cannellini beans, 1 can (15 oz), drained

black beans, 1 can (15 oz) drained

corn, 1 can (15 oz) drained

avocado, 1, chopped

red onion, ¼ of a whole, chopped

roasted red peppers, 1/4 cup, chopped

olive oil, extra virgin, 3 tablespoons

cilantro, fresh, 1 handful, chopped

red wine vinegar, 3 tablespoons

lemon, juice of 1/2

sea salt and pepper to taste

To prepare

1 Combine all ingredients and eat immediately, or chill and serve later. Bon Appetit!

Summer Recipes
Grilled Green Beans

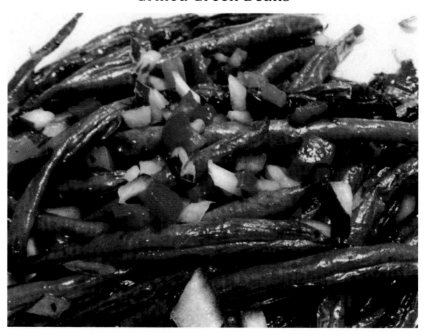

For something new to do with green beans, throw them on the grill. Make sure to buy some extra because you'll lose a couple through the grates. You can use a grilling basket but I like to take my chances.

Green beans are in season late spring and throughout summer. This is when they are at their peak flavor and nutrition. Sometimes I buy haricot verts, if they're local and available. They are a French variety that are smaller, and more delicate in flavor.

Besides the freshest green beans, the secret to this dish is using the best quality olive oil and balsamic vinegar you can find. For a twist, replace the vinegar with fresh squeezed lemon.

Grilled Green Beans

Serves 3 - 5

What you'll need

fresh green beans or haricot verts, 1 bag

red onion, ½ of whole, chopped

roasted red peppers, 3 chopped

olive oil, extra virgin, 2 tablespoons

balsamic vinegar, 2 tablespoons

salt & pepper to taste

To prepare

1 Preheat grill. Wash the green beans and cut off ends.

2 Chop red onion and set aside.

3 Toss green beans with 1 tablespoon of oil & vinegar, salt and pepper.

4 Grill the green beans over medium heat for 4-5 minutes and turn over. Cook for another few minutes turning over occasionally to grill all sides. Remove from heat and toss with red onions and remaining oil and vinegar. Serve warm. Bon Appetit!

Summer Recipes

Fig, Prosciutto, Gorgonzola Pizza - Oven or Grill

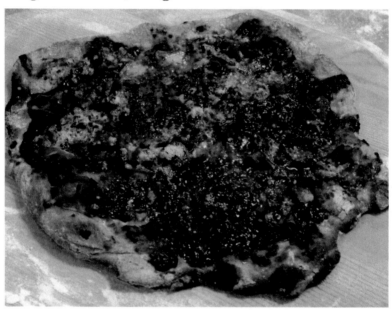

Sweet figs, salty prosciutto and rich gorgonzola on a crispy, charred whole wheat crust equals perfection.

Grilling pizza is fast, easy and absolutely delicious with countless variations. You can make it in the oven as well. Which ingredients do you love? Toss them on. I let my kids choose their ingredients and help assemble their masterpieces. The secret is fresh ingredients, light on the cheese and sauce and a super thin, crispy crust.

Other great pizza toppings

- fresh mozzarella (not the processed kind)
- sausage; chicken or pork
- fresh spinach or sautéed mushrooms
- caramelized onions
- roasted peppers

Fig, Prosciutto, Gorgonzola Pizza - Oven or Grill

One 4 ounce dough serves 1-2

What you'll need

whole wheat dough (get it from your local pizzeria or healthy grocery store, or make it yourself)

prosciutto, several slices, chopped

fresh or dried figs, sliced, chopped, or whole

gorgonzola cheese, crumbled, couple of ounces

pizza stone (for oven)

To prepare

1 Bring the dough to room temperature (it's easier to work with).

2 On a well-floured pizza peel, roll the dough out as thin as possible with a rolling pin, using flour to prevent sticking.

Grill

3 Preheat your grill on medium. Spray the grill with olive oil and gently and carefully transfer the dough onto the grill. Cook for 2-3 minutes, until firm on bottom, then take off the heat, set aside and repeat with remaining dough. Don't cook the other side yet.

4 Position the dough grilled side facing up. Put on the ingredients, starting with the figs, prosciutto, and then the cheese.

5 Place the pie on the grill and cook for 7-10 minutes checking to see when the crust is crispy, removing it when it's charred, not burned. Slice and serve. Bon Appetit!

Oven

3 Place the pizza stone on a middle rack in the oven and preheat to 500 degrees F.

4 Place the ingredients on the dough, starting with the figs, prosciutto, and cheese. Transfer the pie onto the hot pizza stone in the oven. Cook for 5 – 8 minutes, removing when the crust is charred. Slice and serve. Bon Appetit!

Summer Recipes

Fish in a Pouch

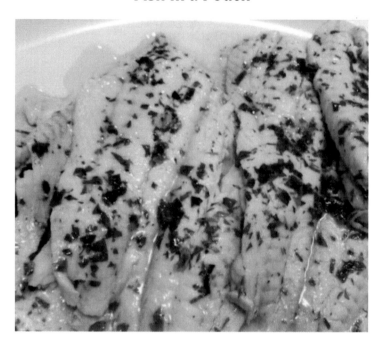

I try to get my kids to eat more fish. It helps to present the fish in interesting ways. This can work for adults who are fish-phobic as well. Try this fish baked in a special package, either using aluminum foil or parchment paper.

Look for wild fish because it seems to have the most health benefits and will not contain antibiotics, which are fed to some farmed fish. I feel more comfortable serving my family a wild fish, living in harmony with nature, than one that's been artificially farmed in unnatural conditions. Some studies show no health difference between the two, but sometimes we should rely on instinct and common sense, rather than lab results.

Befriend your local fishmonger

Find a local fish store and get to know the owner. Ask where they get their fish from; is it wild or farm raised. If it's farmed are they fed antibiotics, or are they grown in a sustainable way? Support local businesses.

Fish in a Pouch

Serves 3-5

What you'll need

fish, 3-4 pounds of your favorite. I like to use Dover sole, which is similar to flounder, but even more mild and sweet in my opinion.

thyme, parsley, oregano, dill, about 1 tablespoon fresh, 1 teaspoon dried

lemon, juice of one large, and more for final squeeze over finished dish

olive oil, extra virgin, 2 tablespoons, and more for drizzling

salt & pepper to taste

Tip: you can also use a splash of your favorite white wine

To prepare

1 Preheat oven to 375. Lay out double layer length of aluminum foil or parchment paper about 24 in long. That's the typical length of a large cutting board.

2 Place the fish, starting in the middle, side by side, trying not to overlap.

3 In a small mixing bowl add herbs, oil, lemon, salt & pepper and wine if you're using. Pour over the fish, trying to cover as much as possible. Fold foil to make a tight little package. You want to try to seal the edges well so the fish steams and the juices remain inside.

4 Place the package on a baking sheet and pop into the hot oven. It will probably take at least 15 minutes for thinner fish, and up to 25 for thicker fish to be done. When you think it's done, take it out, carefully open the package away your face so the escaping steam doesn't burn you and check for doneness. The fish should easily flake and looked uniformly cooked through. Serve as is or transfer to a platter, adding a squeeze of lemon, and drizzle of oil. Bon Appetit!

Serving suggestion: I serve my fish with herb roasted potatoes and softly boiled dandelion greens with lemon and olive oil. It gets rave reviews from the peanut gallery.

Summer Recipes

Skirt Steak over Garden Greens
with Tahini and Hot Sauce

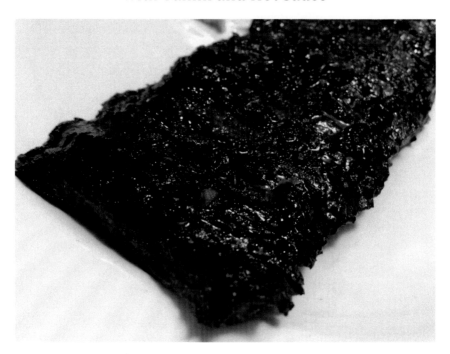

Do you like beef but worry about the health effects of eating beef? I do too. That's why I choose grass-fed beef and bison for it's flavor, health benefit, and sustainability.

I made this dish after a long day working. I craved beef but also wanted to keep the portion small so I served a 4 oz (size of my palm) serving of steak over a Mediterranean salad.

Tahini is a paste made of sesame seeds that can be found in most grocery stores. It's ubiquitous in Greek, Turkish, North African and Middle Eastern Cultures. In this recipe it helps to create a rich creamy dressing that enhances both, greens and animal protein. I love to drizzle it over salads, dip roasted chicken into it, and lace it with a dash of hot sauce like Tabasco or Frank's Red Hot.

Skirt Steak over Garden Greens with Tahini and Hot Sauce

Serves 3-5

What you'll need

skirt steak, grass-fed, 3 – 5 ounces per person, you can also use flank, hanger, or your favorite cut

romaine lettuce, 4 cups or 2 large handfuls

heirloom tomato, 1, cut into 1 inch cubes

onion, ¼ of a small, sliced into thin disks

pickles sliced like matchsticks

sea salt & pepper to taste

Tahini Dressing

tahini, 1 tablespoon

garlic, 1 clove, crushed or finely chopped

lemon, 1 teaspoon or more

water, 2-3 tablespoons

sea salt, pinch

To prepare

1   Remove meat from refrigerator and bring to room temperature. Preheat grill to medium.

2   Chop lettuce, tomato, onions, and pickles and arrange in salad bowl.

3   Grill steak 3-4 minutes on each side for medium rare. Remove from grill and let stand 10 minutes. Slice into strips or squares and place over salad ingredients. Drizzle tahini over salad and enjoy. Bon Appetit

Tahini Dressing

1 Combine tahini, garlic, lemon juice, water, and salt, blend well.

Fall Recipes

Apple Cider, Maple Syrup Vinaigrette over Fall Greens

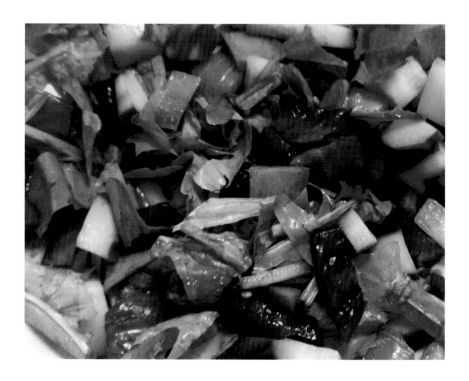

Apples are best in the fall, and that's when I recommend trying this dressing. I serve it over fall greens like arugula, kale, spinach or chard, with apples from the farm, and carrots from the garden. You can try another variation with cranberries and sunflower seeds.

I recommend real maple syrup, not the fake stuff with processed sugars and additives.

And use a good quality Dijon mustard without additives or preservatives to make your dressings and marinades.

Apple Cider, Maple Syrup Vinaigrette
over Fall Greens

Serves 3 - 5

What You'll Need

apple cider vinegar, ¼ cup

red onion, or shallot, 2 tablespoons, chopped fine

olive oil, extra virgin, 2 tablespoons

maple syrup, 1 tablespoon

Dijon mustard, 1 tablespoon

sea salt & pepper to taste

Greens

Try fall arugula, spinach, kale, chard, or romaine, 2 large handfuls, chopped

How To Prepare

1 Chop the shallot or onion and toss in a bowl with the vinegar, maple syrup, and mustard and stir.

2 Slowly pour in the olive oil while whisking. Serve over greens salad.

Tips - Make extra dressing and store in the fridge for a week.

Typically, I use red onions for salads & dressings, yellow onions for cooking, and Vidalia or Spanish onions for grilling.

Fall Recipes

Garlic Roasted Brussels Sprouts

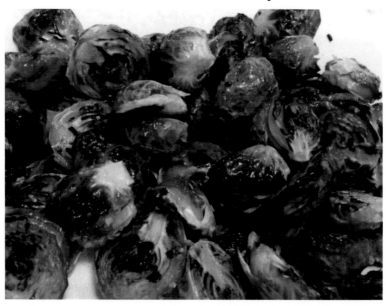

Years ago I worked for a chiropractor that would rave about his roasted Brussels sprouts; garlicky, charred, lightly salted, tender but toothy. He made them sound so appealing I had to try them. I did, and I was hooked. This is his simple recipe that I've been using ever since.

Tips: Use flavored salt from a gourmet market; smoked, garlic, herbed, truffle.

Drizzle on the best quality olive oil you can find before serving.

Eat vegetables in their own season for the best flavor and nutrition.

Fall veggies: Brussels sprouts, broccoli, broccoli rabe, beets, cabbage, cauliflower, leeks, parsnips, carrots

Garlic Roasted Brussels Sprouts

Serves 3 - 5

What You'll Need

Brussels sprouts, 1 pound

garlic, 2-3 cloves

olive oil, extra virgin, 3-4 tablespoons

sea salt to taste

To prepare

1 Preheat oven to 400 degrees. Wash Brussels Sprouts, cut off stem end, slice in half, remove outer leaves and drop into a large bowl.

2 Peel and finely chop the garlic, scoop into bowl. Drizzle with olive oil and sprinkle to salt.

3 Roll out onto a large baking sheet lined with parchment paper, and pop into the oven.

4 Check them after 7-10 minutes, and flip when they're browned on the bottom. Cook for another 7-10 minutes, and remove when they are charred and fork tender. Don't overcook; you want them al dente, (a little firm but done). Serve immediately in a large bowl with another drizzle of oil and pinch of salt. Bon Appetit!

Tip

If they're almost done but not yet browned, put them under the broiler to crisp them up a bit.

Fall Recipes

Autumn Beet and Grape Salad

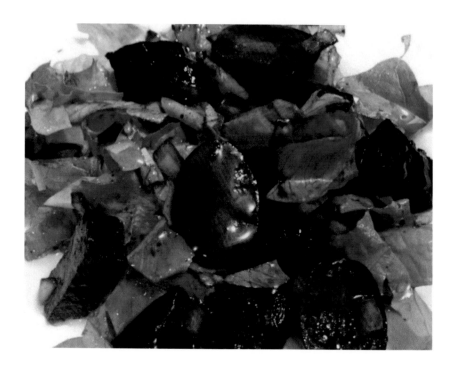

Beets are popular again and for good reason. They're delicious in salads and at their best in the fall. If you hated them as a child there's a good chance it was because they came out of a can. Forget the can; grow them, get them at the farmers market, or buy them precooked, just not in a can.

I picked mine up at my local organic farm. The sweetness and crunch of the grapes are a nice compliment, and contrast to the earthy softness of the beets. I also used salad greens from my greenhouse garden.

They also come in different colors, which liven up any dish with flavor and good nutrition.

Autumn Beet and Grape Salad

Serves 4-5

What You'll Need

beets, 2-3, or a package of pre-cooked (they're so easy to make, I recommend fresh)

grapes, red or green, 1 cup

salad greens, 4 - 5 cups, I used a fancy gourmet blend

red onion, 1/4 of a medium, chopped

balsamic vinegar, 2 tablespoons, (use a good quality vinegar)

olive oil, extra virgin, 3 tablespoons

sea salt & pepper to taste

To prepare

1 If you're roasting the beets: Preheat the oven to 400 degrees. Wash and wrap the beets in foil, place on a cooking sheet, and cook for 1 hour, or until fork tender. Remove and let cool.

2 Wash and slice the grapes in half. Chop the red onion fine and place both in a mixing bowl. Wash and coarsely chop the lettuce and arrange in a salad bowl.

3 When the beets have cooled, put 1 plastic baggy on each hand, like gloves, and peel the outer layer of the beets off. The thin skin should remove easily. You do this because the beets color everything they touch red. Slice the beets and then chop into ½ inch cubes.

4 Place the beets in the bowl with the grapes and onions, drizzle in the olive oil and vinegar and season with salt and pepper. Toss, gently arrange over the greens, and serve. Bon Appetit!

Fall Recipes

Acorn Squash Soup

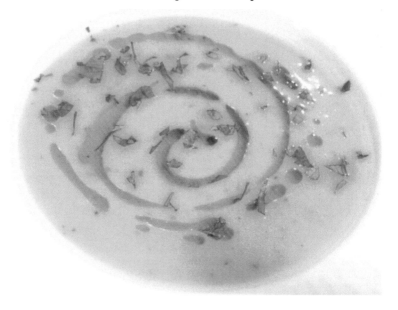

Does anything say fall more than a squash soup, aside from an apple pie. The acorn squash is so impossibly sweet; this dish becomes a warm, savory autumn meal, served simply with a warm beet salad. Perfection.

Squash tips

Ask your grocer to peel and chop them for you.

If you cut your own, use a very sharp knife and vegetable peeler, and work in small sections.

Have a fear of pasta carbs? Try spaghetti squash for a delicious alternative to pasta.

When pureed, you'll swear this dish has heavy cream, but it doesn't. In fact, it's vegan, with full flavor and satisfaction.

Acorn Squash Soup

Serves 3 – 5 with leftovers for the freezer

What You'll Need

> *acorn squash, 2 medium*
>
> *potatoes, yukon or red, 4 small*
>
> *carrots, 2 medium*
>
> *onions, 1 medium*
>
> *garlic, 2 cloves*
>
> *vegetable broth, or water, 5 cups*
>
> *water, 3 cups*
>
> *olive oil, extra virgin*
>
> *nutmeg, grated fresh, 1 teaspoon*
>
> *sea salt & pepper to taste*
>
> *thyme, fresh, 2 sprigs, or 1 tablespoon*
>
> *parsley, fresh, 1 tablespoon, and some for garnish*

To prepare

1 Preheat oven to 400 degrees. Wash and cut the squash top and bottom off (careful, the skin is thick). Scoop out the seeds with a spoon, cut into chunks, drizzle with olive oil and place on a baking sheet. Cook for 35 - 45 minutes, until the flesh easily forks.

2 Peel and chop the onion, carrots, and potatoes. In a large Dutch oven or heavy pot over medium heat, add about 4 tablespoons of olive oil. Add the onions and sauté for 5 minutes, then add the rest of the vegetables. Crush the garlic and add. Sauté for another 10 minutes. If the acorn squash is not done, turn off heat and set aside.

3 Remove the squash from the oven and add to the pot. Add the broth, season generously with salt, and lightly pepper. Bring to a boil, turn to a low simmer, and cook for 20 minutes. Using a stick blender, or blender, puree till smooth and thick. Ladle into a bowl, drizzle with olive oil, parsley and serve. Bon Appetit!

Fall Recipes

Braised, Pastured Lamb Shanks

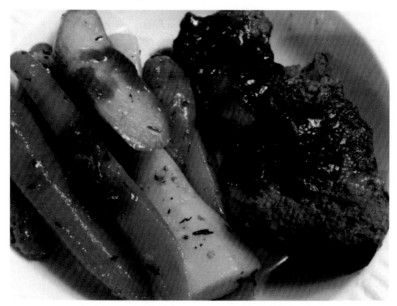

This lamb melts at the site of a fork. Just allow plenty of cooking time, like 6 hours, and worth every one of them. The longer this dish cooks, the more flavor you get.

I'm convinced that if someone doesn't like lamb, they've never had it prepared correctly. My family, including my kids, are now lamb lovers thanks to this dish. We serve it with potatoes and carrots. *(See Gourmet French Vegetables recipe on page 18)*

Tips: I used pastured (grass fed) lamb, from my local healthy market. Pastured animals can roam, eat traditional foods, and are healthier than conventionally raised animals. They containing more omega-3s, are leaner, and sustainably raised.

I recommend buying American, local lamb, as opposed to Australian or New Zealand, which can taste more gamey and had to fly thousands of miles to get to your plate. My favorite cuts are shanks braised, a leg roasted, and chops and shoulders grilled.

Braised, Pastured Lamb Shanks

Serves 5 with leftovers (I used 5 lamb shanks)

What You'll Need

> *lamb, shanks or shoulder steaks, 1 per person*
>
> *onion, 1 large, chopped fine*
>
> *carrots, 3, chopped fine*
>
> *celery, 3 stalks, chopped fine*
>
> *garlic, 3-5 cloves, crushed*
>
> *tomatoes, stewed, 28 oz can (I use certified San Marzano)*
>
> *red wine, or port, 1 bottle*
>
> *thyme, rosemary, oregano, about 3 sprigs fresh, or 3 tablespoons each, or 1 tablespoon each dried*
>
> *olive oil, extra virgin, 4-5 tablespoons*
>
> *sea salt & pepper to taste (I'm generous with the salt)*
>
> *good bread for dipping!*

How To Prepare

1 Preheat the oven to 250 degrees, placing rack in the middle. In a large, heavy-duty pot, I use a Le Creuset Dutch Oven, heat 2 tablespoons of the oil over medium high heat. When the oil is hot, brown the lamb on all sides. (Don't salt the lamb or it will draw out water and prevent it from browning.) Take your time with this and don't crowd the meat or it will steam instead of brown.

2 Meanwhile, finely chop the onion, carrots, celery, and crush the garlic. When the lamb is browned, remove to a plate, pour in the rest of the olive oil and sauté the onions over low heat for 10 minutes. Then add the carrots, celery and garlic, sauté for 5 more minutes.

3 Add the tomatoes to the pot, crushing them in your palm and through your fingers. Pour in the wine, and toss in the herb sprigs, or chop them and add. Add the lamb with its juices.

4 Bring to a gentle pre-boil (burping bubbles), and immediately place in the oven, covered. Check occasionally and give it a stir. Remove after 6 hours (It's probably done after 2 hours, but 6 is when the magic happens), let sit for at least 30 minutes, covered. Serve with carrots and potatoes, or a favorite grain like orzo, or quinoa, or over mashed potatoes or turnips. Bon Appetit!

Resources

I use these resources to help me shop, cook, and eat healthy.

Food Shopping

Local Farms: *localharvest.org/organic-farms/*

Farmers Markets: *localharvest.org/farmers-markets/*

Whole Foods: *wholefoodsmarket.com/stores/list*

Trader Joes: *traderjoes.com/*

Greensbury Market: A modern day online market offering organic, sustainably raised beef, pork, and poultry from small farms, and sustainably harvested seafood. *greensburymarket.com*

Local Butchers, Bakers, Seafood Markets, Farm to Table Restaurants

Organic Gardening

Elliot Coleman: A pioneer in the modern organic farm movement. He'll teach you everything about home gardening. I recommend all of his books as quintessential resources. *fourseasonfarm.com*

Johnny's Seeds: large selection of organic gardening seeds. *johnnyseeds.com*

Recipes

Food and Wine Magazine – Recipes are shared by professional chefs and tested for the home kitchen. I "healthify" them, typically by replacing butter with olive oil, white pasta with whole grain, reducing the sodium, and so on. *foodandwine.com*

Food Network: I like to source my recipes from professional chefs and then modify them to my family's liking; making them healthier and using fresh, local, seasonal ingredients. *foodnetwork.com/recipes.html*

Jacques Pepin: Is world-renowned as a chef and the host of his acclaimed and popular cooking programs on public television, and as a respected instructor, a prolific author and gifted artist. He is my go to source for all things cooking. *blogs.kqed.org/essentialpepin*

Cooking Tips

foodandwine.com/jacques-pepin-cooking-videos

How to Read Food Labels

1. Look at the ingredients - The first ingredient should be the food it is. If the first ingredient is sugar, think twice. If it's a grain, look for "whole". If you can't pronounce it, move on.

2. Check the sugar content. Look for 10 grams of sugar or less per serving

3. Buy foods that come without a food label – think fruit, vegetables, bulk grains, nuts, seeds, and animal products in their whole, or recognizable state (unprocessed).

More tips

- Avoid trans fats, hydrogenated oils, high fructose corn syrup and other artificial and processed additives
- Sodium per serving - look for 120 mg or less of sodium per serving or 5 % DV (Percent Daily Value).
- Dietary fiber greater than 1 gram per serving.

Index

C

4